ESSENTIAL WISDOM

Overcoming the Barriers to a Healthy, Happy, and Balanced Life

Esperanza Granados-Bezi

Dedication

To my son Oscar Didier, my dearest treasure, and the greatest inspiration in every endeavor. With love forever.

To my husband Octavio Oscar, the best companion to share this wonderful journey of life.

To everyone I know who struggles to achieve long-lasting health and happiness.

Acknowledgment

I would like to thank my beloved brother Gerardo for being the second pillar behind this book. I am grateful for his never-ending patience, unconditional technical support, and faith in my various projects.

This book was made possible by the collaboration of a generous and bright group of people who reviewed my drafts, providing insightful suggestions to improve them. I am especially indebted to my friend David Lorenzatti who has been proofreading my texts for many years. He has read and revised many sections of this manuscript, giving high-quality, thoughtful feedback and great ideas with diligence.

About the Author

Esperanza Granados- Bezi Ph.D is a professor, researcher, and speaker in the areas of Education, Health, and Wellness. She believes that the most urgent responsibility every person has is to keep their body and mind in optimal condition throughout life. Since she is convinced that achieving good health is in our hands, she has become an advocate for the development of healthy habits that promote long-lasting well-being and prevent chronic diseases.

Table of Contents

Introduction

It is a common belief that our genetic code and personal circumstances determine the quality of our life and the level of our well-being. However, the daily decisions we make concerning nutrition, exercise, relationships, education, finances, and other practical matters, can have an even greater impact on how balanced and fulfilling our life can be. Genes do not determine our destiny; we do. Our decisions, actions, and thoughts are what shape our future. We can choose to rise above our genetics and create a life of our own design.

I am convinced that, even though we may not be able to change every aspect of ourselves or our world, most people can design the kind of existence they desire. Indeed, we can become the architects of our destinies once we realize that our attitudes and habits may improve or damage our health and happiness. We can also foster resilience to recover from personal trauma, overcome substance abuse, or control our weight, among other things. It takes courage and good judgement to be able to push through hard times, and resilience can provide us with the support to do just that. With resilience, we can find the strength to start anew and reach our goals.

But developing good judgment does not entail becoming experts in psychology, medicine, or philosophy. The secret to leading fulfilling and successful lives lies in gaining or increasing our wisdom to adopt behaviors that can lead to healthier and balanced lifestyles.

Wisdom has been defined as the ability to achieve meaningful lives by making sensible and rational decisions. It is related to cultivating sound judgment to overcome life's challenges and seeking alternatives to move forward. Wisdom allows people to apply knowledge effectively, adapt to life changes, learn from past experiences, and seek help and support. Learning what is best for us is not enough. We must make every effort to put that knowledge into action.

While education and experience contribute to increased wisdom, they do not guarantee that a person has become wiser. Having information leads to wisdom when knowledge promotes personal fulfillment and joy. On the other hand, experiences increase our wisdom when we reflect on them and they help us better understand ourselves, others, and our circumstances.

The main components of wisdom are a realistic approach to life; making good life choices; the ability to solve problems and to evaluate the risks and consequences of one's actions; a capacity to learn from previous mistakes; a sensibility to identify and modify flaws and habits that harm us; and a willingness to accept constructive criticism or advice from caring individuals. Wisdom is usually associated with prudence, caution, awareness, responsibility, discipline, integrity, patience, and gratitude.

As a first step in increasing my wisdom, I began researching effective strategies to achieve long-lasting well-being. One of the first lessons I learned was that leading a life of good health and vitality has more to do with how we choose to live and less with our circumstances. Thus, we must learn to treat ourselves with care and kindness because adopting detrimental or self-destructive behaviors will make us sick, empty, and unhappy.

Although we live in times of unprecedented scientific research, some people take their physical, mental, and emotional health for granted. They continue to develop habits that only make them comfortable or that might bring short-term gratification, regardless of the impact on their well-being. They usually forget that our body and brain are extraordinary treasures given to us in excellent condition so that we can enjoy our journey and fulfill our potential.

I recently moved to an active senior community where I have seen firsthand the consequences of personal choices in how we live and age. Observing some of my neighbors have made it evident how our daily habits help us defy the laws of time or lead to the early deterioration of our bodies and minds. I have encountered middle-aged people who have trouble performing regular daily activities due to excessive weight or a sedentary lifestyle. Fortunately, I have also met many fit, healthy, autonomous seniors in their eighties and nineties who are fully engaged with peers and continue enjoying their retirement years.

Aging is unavoidable, but how we act in our youth and adult life will allow us to enjoy our golden years or turn us into frail, physically disabled, and even mentally challenged individuals. Consequently, our most urgent responsibility is to keep our body and mind in optimal condition at every stage of life. Self-care is crucial to long-lasting well-being.

In my quest for wisdom, I have discovered many valuable ideas for living life positively. At the same time, I have discovered a vocation for encouraging people to become the best version of themselves. Regardless of age, we all need guidance and support to learn to live well, grow and thrive.

The purpose of this book is to persuade readers that we all need to foster good living experiences. It contains useful principles you can apply to your circumstances to help you live a well-balanced life. We all have access to books and other widely circulated publications promoting healthy living principles. However, reviewing these resources can be time-consuming and overwhelming, given the contradictory approaches and misinformation we sometimes encounter.

Early in my career as an educator, I learned that information should be presented concisely and simplified so that it can be easily understood, remembered, and put into practice. On the other hand, as a passionate advocate for long-lasting wellness, I can attest that the strategies discussed in this text have helped me age gracefully and that they can also benefit you and others to successfully reach optimal health and enjoy the rewarding outcomes of longevity and fitness.

Your interest in this book demonstrates that you are ready to explore the sources of positive physical, mental, emotional, and spiritual practices. The book can be read in a sequence, from the first chapter to the last, or you can select chapters randomly. Please read my observations and suggestions and use the book as a reference. It will lead you on a journey along the path to a healthier and more satisfying lifestyle.

Moreover, because this book has also been designed as a companion guide on your path to better health, I recommend incorporating the information provided into your life routines. Knowledge only becomes wisdom when we put it into practice. This is the best way to take responsibility for achieving optimal health. The first step in that direction begins with doing some reflective work and providing specific answers to the questions at the end of each chapter.

Book's Principles:

· Genetics or life's circumstances do not fully control our destiny; our actions, habits, and decisions majorly impact our physical, mental, and emotional well-being.

· Most people can transform their lives by increasing their wisdom, changing their mindsets, modifying unhealthy behaviors, or overcoming addictions.

· Wisdom is the ability to achieve meaningful and fulfilling lives by cultivating sound judgment, which allows us to make sensible and smart decisions.

· Smart decisions result from increasing and internalizing knowledge, developing self-awareness, learning from mistakes, and accepting positive criticism.

· The value we place on ourselves is reflected in our self-esteem, which has a direct impact on the choices we make every day.

· Today's choices can bring us closer to the best version of ourselves or determine the number of regrets we have tomorrow, in five years, or for the rest of our lives.

· Wise people practice self-care and do not neglect or mistreat their bodies with self-destructive behaviors like overeating, substance abuse, reckless driving, etc.

· Every person needs guidance, inspiration, and support in the process of developing the wisdom that can lead to a well-balanced life.

· When self-care becomes a priority in our life, we make the best investment in ourselves and our happiness because no possession is as precious as our health.

· Keeping our body and mind in optimal condition requires discipline and sacrifice but living free of physical, mental, and emotional pain is the most rewarding benefit.

· Aging is unavoidable, but self-care at every stage of life leads to long-lasting well-being, preventing chronic diseases, disability, and premature death.

· Optimal health and well-being are essential for achieving satisfying, productive, and successful lives.

· Regardless of the current condition of our health, recovery is possible with the right attitude, an adequate approach, and caring support.

· Change only happens when we are determined to adopt a healthier lifestyle, prioritize these efforts, and commit to the hard work needed for success.

Chapter 1:

Dimensions of Wellness

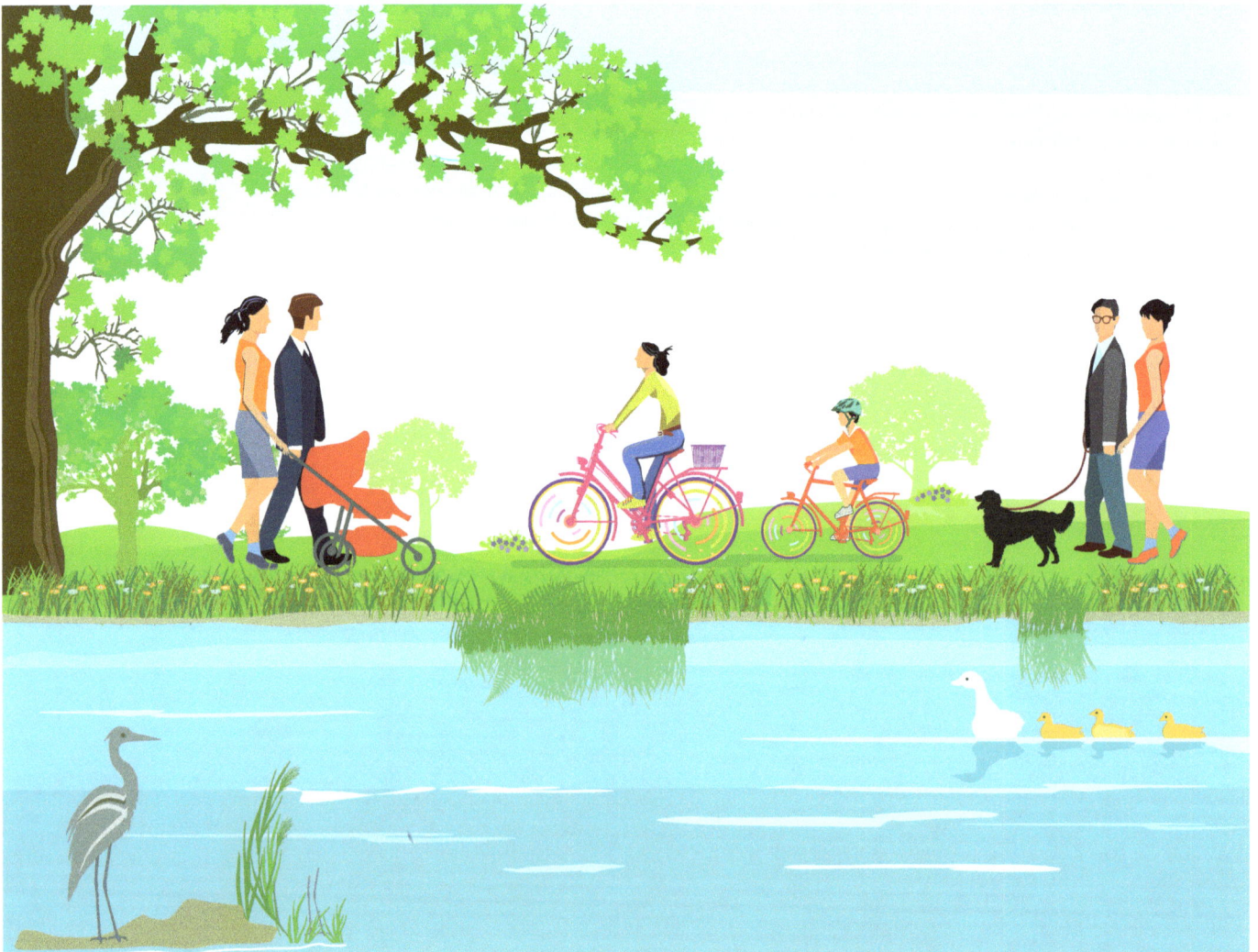

The World Health Organization states that good health is "a state of complete physical and emotional well-being." Physical wellness involves developing a lifestyle that enhances health and prevents injuries and illness. Mental wellness is maintaining a balanced psychological, social, and emotional life.

Our body and mind must be nourished and kept finely tuned for many reasons. First, a healthy body and mind allow us to feel motivated and energized to face life's challenges, responsibilities, and pleasures daily. Second, they are essential to lead an active, productive, and meaningful life. Third, we start to age from birth, and our genes may predispose us to develop certain diseases.

From a medical point of view, there are two types of aging: regular and successful. Regular aging is the natural process where our bodies and minds start to deteriorate with time. This process is unavoidable and leaves people more vulnerable to diseases and injury as they age. On the other hand, successful aging is when a person can maintain physical and mental health at a high level even as they age. While regular aging is unavoidable and affects everyone, successful aging is a process that can be managed and improved.

Successful aging is achieved through healthy lifestyle habits, mental stimulation, and physical activity. Eating a balanced diet, exercising regularly, and getting enough sleep are all essential to successful aging. Additionally, mental stimulation is important for keeping the brain active and healthy and can be achieved through activities like puzzle games and reading. Regular physical activity also helps to reduce the risk of diseases and injuries and can help maintain independence in older adults. Successful aging is being physically and mentally sharp well into the 80s and 90s. (There are about 125 million people older than 80 in the world today, and there will be about 450 million by 2050.)

Our physical health is determined by various factors such as body mass index (BMI,) fitness, nutrition, and sleep habits. (BMI is a formula that provides a numerical rating of our health based on weight and height.) A healthy body is not perfect or ideal but represents our best self at any age. It allows us to thrive, free of degenerating diseases, pain, and addictions. It may not be possible for everyone to avoid getting sick completely, but we must take responsibility for preventing injuries and illness, regardless of age.

Mental health is associated with a person's ability to enjoy life, manage stress, keep strong relationships, and develop a sense of purpose. Good mental health helps us to make the most of our lives and cope with adversity and challenges. It can help us to have a positive outlook on life and be resilient in the face of difficult times. It is manifested in our capacity to live in peace and harmony with ourselves and the world around us. A healthy mind is not affected by disorders, such as excessive tension, anxiety, frustration, anger, and depression. Therefore, taking steps to ensure our mental health is taken care of is essential for living a life of balance and fulfillment.

Many health professionals believe that about half of what affects our health is determined by our life choices and that the essential factors to aging well are within each person's control. For instance, having regular medical checkups can help someone detect a disease before it fully develops, thus preventing early death.

The National Institute of Health and the World Health Organization support that if more people stopped smoking, lost weight, and exercised regularly, about 80% of heart disease, stroke, and diabetes and 40% of cancers could be prevented. Our actions have a direct impact on improving or worsening an ailment. For this reason, being mindful of our decisions and willing to make necessary behavioral changes will certainly result in dramatic lifespan increases.

If any part of our body is significantly harmed, it can be very hard, if not impossible, to fix it. This can negatively impact our lives. People who care for themselves do not abuse their bodies, such as through excessive eating or engaging in drug use. Additionally, they do not participate in dangerous activities that could be detrimental to their health, like speeding, casual sexual encounters, or intense sports, as these can often result in early death.

Keeping our body and mind in the best condition requires discipline and sacrifices, but living free of physical and emotional pain, or discomfort is highly rewarding. We must learn to modify our habits, especially the compulsive behaviors that interfere with our capacity to make well-thought-out choices that sidetrack our progress toward a healthier lifestyle. Once we experience and enjoy the benefits of being healthy and fit, we will not want to neglect our body and mind again.

We all have different health needs, bodies and minds, and living circumstances. Thus, optimal well-being might be different for each person, and the path to achieving wellness may also vary from one person to another. However, the foundations of a healthy lifestyle are universal, requiring us to learn to enjoy life's joys with moderation. Ah, and the sooner we start protecting our body, the higher our chances of living in better health and longer.

A vital step in the path to healthier living starts with becoming more knowledgeable about the principles of wellness and the best ways to prevent disease. This understanding should force us to identify the behaviors that benefit or harm our health. After we decide which areas need improvement, we must put the recommendations given by experts into practice.

An important recommendation I can give you before you continue reading this book is that spending time, effort, and some money to create the healthiest version of yourself is the best investment you can ever make because no possession is as precious as your health! Moreover, accept that you alone have the power to control your destiny and that you will also be the one who benefits the most from your wellness wisdom.

- A healthy body and mind are essential to lead an active, productive, and meaningful life.

- A healthy mind is free from tension, anxiety, frustration, anger, and depression.

- Positive behavioral changes will increase your well-being and prevent chronic diseases.

- It is very difficult or almost impossible to fix or replace severely damaged organs.

Questions to reflect on

1. When you look at yourself in a mirror, does it reflect your best-self for your age? (Explain)

2. What is needed in your life for you to feel physically and mentally healthier?

3. Based on that information, what are the two most urgent behavioral changes that you need to undertake?

Chapter 2:

Understanding Key Nutritional Concepts and Calorie Intake

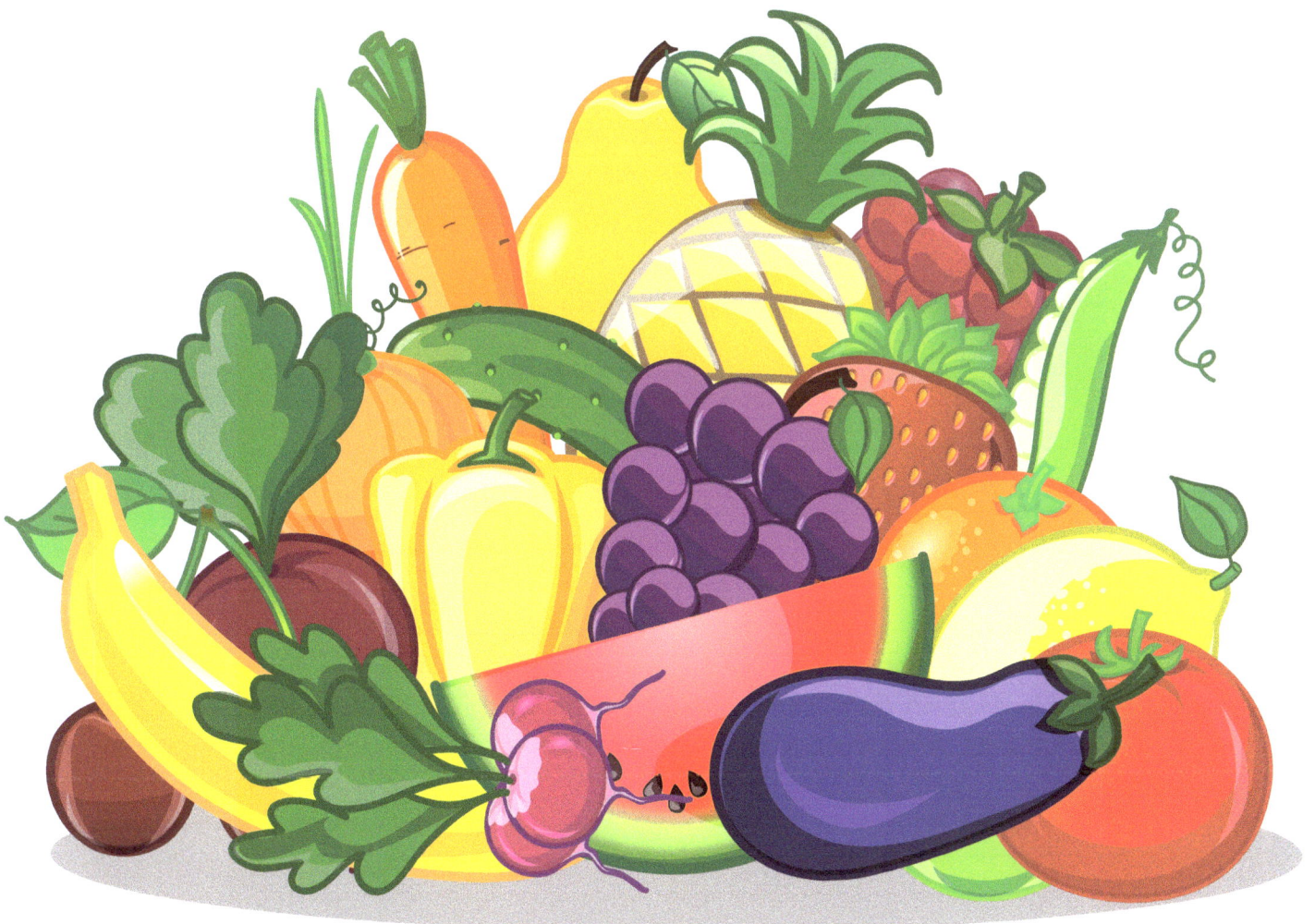

Good nutrition and good eating habits are crucial to our well-being. Food should nourish and sustain both our body and our mind. It should provide all the necessary elements for optimal health. In order to develop healthy eating habits, we must understand basic nutritional concepts to guide us in making smart decisions. We may already know some of this information, but it is always useful to review it.

Foods are made of one or many types of essential nutrients: carbohydrates, fats, proteins, vitamins, minerals, and water.

Digestion occurs when nutrients are extracted from food, combined with oxygen (supplied by breathing,) and transformed into chemical nutrients and energy. In general, they break down as follows:

- carbohydrates into simple sugars or glucose

- fats into fatty acids and glycerol

- proteins into amino acids and chemicals from plant-based foods.

Knowing how food is absorbed into the body will help you maintain a balanced diet. It may require limiting or avoiding certain foods while increasing the consumption of others.

I do not believe in disparaging any food group, although I suggest keeping the use of sugar, salt, and alcohol to the minimum. In addition, I firmly believe in the 80/20 rule, which recommends eating healthy foods 80% of the time.

Carbohydrates are the main source of blood glucose, a major fuel for all the body's cells, and the only energy source for the brain and red blood cells. Carbohydrates help maintain energy levels, support sharp mental functions, and replenish starved muscles. However, not all carbs are beneficial to our bodies.

There are two forms of carbohydrates: simple and complex. **Simple carbohydrates** are digested very quickly and immediately released into the bloodstream. They include sugars found naturally in foods such as fruits, vegetables, milk, and dairy products. They are also found in refined or highly processed foods like white bread, white rice, cookies, cakes, pasta, sodas, and sweets.

Most weight loss programs recommend restricting or avoiding simple carbs that are processed or not plant-based because they contain little nutritional value and provide "empty calories." They also trigger a sugar rush, stimulating the immediate release of insulin, but after about an hour, they cause our blood sugar to drop, leaving us hungry, fatigued, or sluggish.

Consuming simple carbs leads you to crave more. High consumption of simple carbohydrates makes your body store them as fat, which can lead to obesity.

Complex carbohydrates have higher nutrient values than simple carbs. They are good sources of fiber, sugar, vitamins, and minerals. They are digested slowly, which makes us feel full and satisfied for much longer.

Carbohydrates should be eaten in their natural, whole, unprocessed form to give us the energy we need and keep our blood sugar levels steady. Complex carbs include whole-grain bread and cereals, starchy vegetables, and legumes. Here is a list of unhealthy and healthy carbs.

Unhealthy Carbs	Healthy Carbs
• Fruit juice concentrate	• Fruits
• Sweet drinks and sodas	• Vegetables
• White rice, pasta, and pizza	• Brown rice and whole-grain pasta
• Baked treats	• Whole grain cereals (oatmeal)
• Candy and ice cream	• Nuts and seeds
• Refined or processed foods	• Beans, soybeans, and lentils

Fats. Although much attention has been given to reducing dietary fat, this macronutrient is essential to provide energy and optimize our health. Fat is the largest source of energy available to the body and the least to stimulate insulin spikes.

Unfortunately, the modern diet includes excessive amounts of fats, primarily from fast and fried foods, contributing to many diseases. Excessive fat intake is a major factor in obesity, high blood pressure, coronary heart disease, and colon cancer. It has been linked to several other disorders as well.

There are healthy and unhealthy fats. Healthy fats (essential fatty acids) are necessary for a well-balanced diet. Essential fatty acids can be found in their healthiest form in high-quality, less processed, non-hydrogenated oils. Healthy oils include extra-virgin olive oil, fish oil, and sesame oil. A diet that includes foods rich in healthy fats will promote excellent mental and physical health.

Saturated and trans fats are considered unhealthy fats for most people. They are difficult to digest and burn to provide energy; they form a plaque in our arteries, increasing triglyceride and bad cholesterol levels. They should be kept to a minimum in our diet or, depending on our health, be avoided completely. Here is a list of unhealthy and healthy fats.

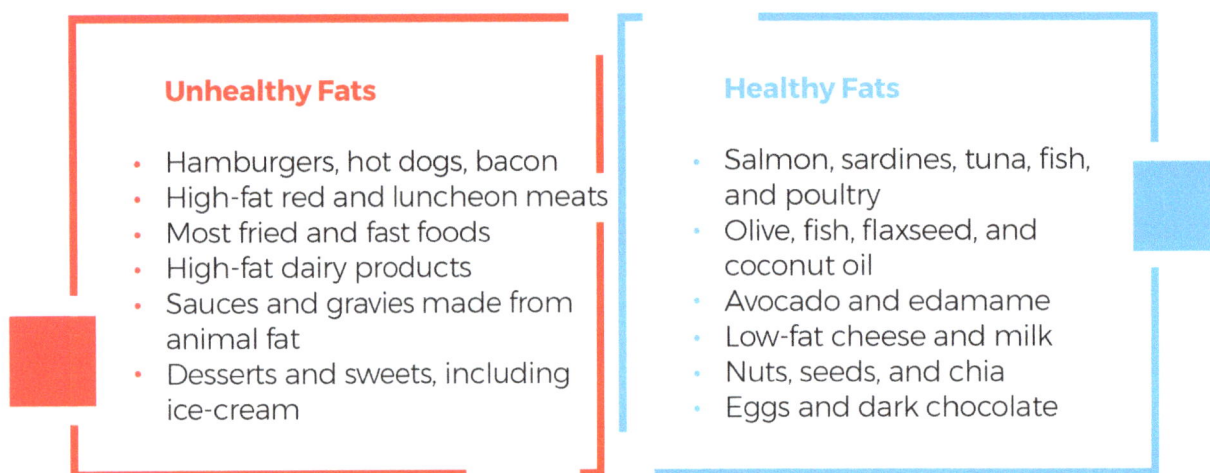

Unhealthy Fats

- Hamburgers, hot dogs, bacon
- High-fat red and luncheon meats
- Most fried and fast foods
- High-fat dairy products
- Sauces and gravies made from animal fat
- Desserts and sweets, including ice-cream

Healthy Fats

- Salmon, sardines, tuna, fish, and poultry
- Olive, fish, flaxseed, and coconut oil
- Avocado and edamame
- Low-fat cheese and milk
- Nuts, seeds, and chia
- Eggs and dark chocolate

Proteins are essential to keep our body running smoothly. They give us long-lasting energy and are needed to produce hormones, antibodies, and enzymes. They also help repair tissues and keep muscles strong. Proteins have hunger-reducing benefits because they are digested slowly, which causes them to remain longer in the digestive tract. Most foods contain some protein, so the sources are abundant.

When protein is consumed, the body breaks it down into amino acids. They can be *nonessential* or *essential*. Nonessential amino acids are not diet specific. Our body can synthesize them from other amino acids. They are found in various foods, including grains, legumes, and leafy green vegetables.

Essential amino acids are diet specific. Proteins produce eight essential amino acids in fish, poultry, meat, cheese, eggs, and milk. Although beef is considered high in saturated fat, it can still be a part of a healthy diet, provided it is grass-fed, lean, and sparingly eaten. But we must avoid processed meats such as bacon, sausages, salami, prosciutto, or other deli meats. They are linked to cancer, diabetes, degenerative diseases, and fatty liver.

Like water, carbohydrates, protein, fats, **vitamins,** and **minerals** are essential to life. However, vitamins and minerals are often called *micronutrients* simply because they are needed in relatively small amounts compared to the three main nutrients.

After reviewing the main food nutrients, let us remember that when it comes to maintaining a healthy body and preventing diseases, the nutrients in our food are our best medicine. In contrast, taking over-the-counter supplements and vitamins can be a tricky practice.

Many of these products come from unregulated industries, and some may even be detrimental to our health. That is because neither the effectiveness nor the safety of supplements and vitamins needs to be proven by research. Therefore, the claims about their benefits may be false, and we may waste our money or compromise our well-being.

Understanding Caloric Intake

Calories. In nutrition, **calories** refer to the energy people get from what they eat and drink and the energy they use in physical activity. The number of daily calories we need depends on age, height, gender, and activity level. Here is a table to help determine the calories we need to meet our energy demands. (Source: Webmed.com)

Recommended Daily Caloric Intake				
Gender	Age	Sedentary	Active	Very Active
Female	9 - 25	1500	1700	2100
	26 - 50	1800	2000	2200
	51 +	1600	1800	2000
Male	9 - 25	1600	1800	2200
	26 - 50	2300	2400	2600
	51 +	2100	2300	2400

Many diets recommend counting calories as a good way to keep track of our food intake; however, doing so can be rather annoying and time-consuming for some people. In my experience, reducing food portions is a better alternative to help me control my weight. I have become accustomed to eating small portions and stop eating once my hunger is satisfied. Normally, the less I eat, the better and more energized I feel.

Regardless of whether we count calories regularly, being aware of the calorie content in the most common foods is an excellent way to remain vigilant about our dietary intake. Here is a list of the calories of some common foods to be used as a quick reference. *(Source: USDA National Nutrient Database for Standard Reference.)*

Fruits (Calories)	
1 Avocado	270
1 Medium mango	107
1 Medium banana	105
1 Medium apple	72
1 Pear	64
Grapes (100 grams)	60
1 Orange	60
Watermelon (1 cup)	46
1 Medium grapefruit	45
Pineapple (2 slices)	40
1 Peach	36
Strawberries (100 grams)	27

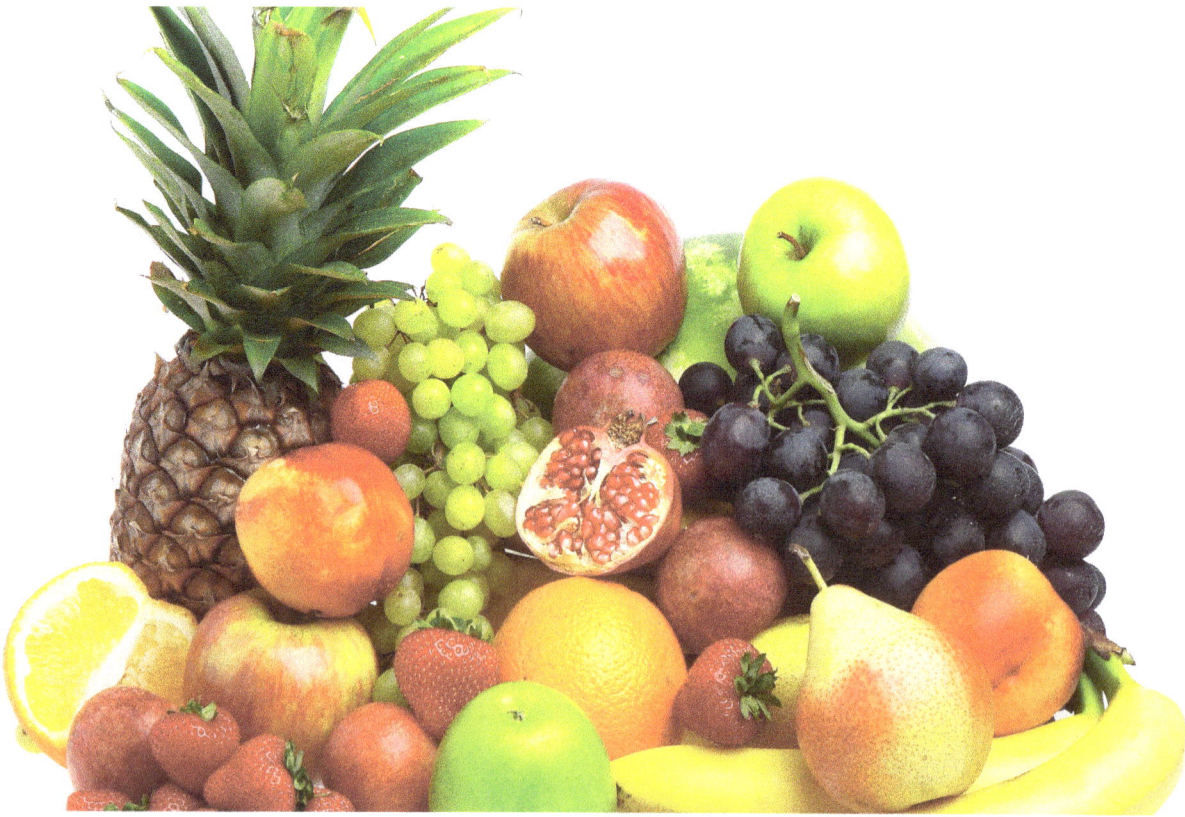

Vegetables (Calories)

Medium French fries	340
Chickpeas (1 cup)	295
Kidney beans (1 cup)	230
1 medium potato	168
Corn (1 cup)	140
Onion (1 cup)	65
Spinach (1 cup)	36
Asparagus (1 cup)	36
Green beans (1 cup)	31
Broccoli (1 cup)	30
1 Cucumber	30
Carrots (1 cup)	30
Cauliflower (1 cup)	28
Mushrooms (1 cup)	20
Celery (3 stalks)	9
Lettuce (1 cup)	7

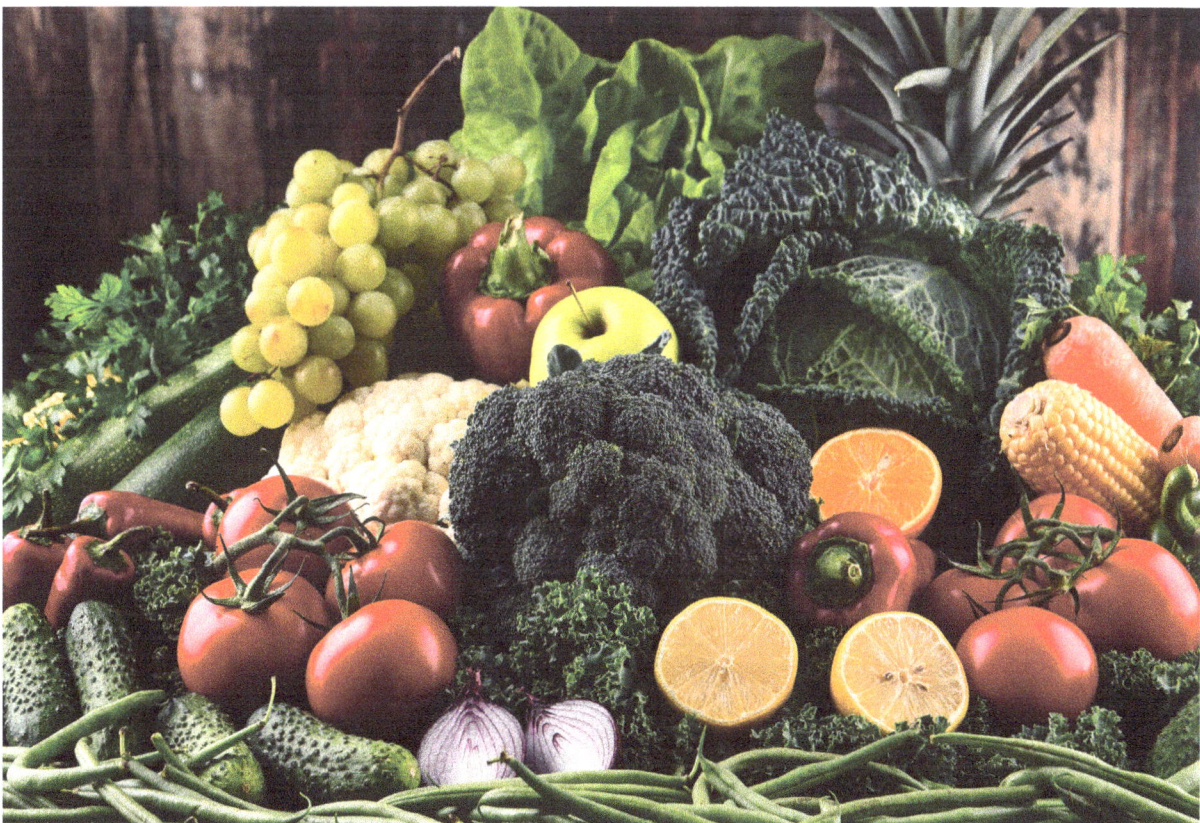

Mixed salads contain good amounts of essential nutrients; however, the total number of calories in a salad depends on the dressing, protein or other added ingredients. A healthy salad becomes less nutritious if you add a rich dressing or fatty ingredients. Also, fast food salads tend to have a very high calorie content. For example:

- A large Caesar salad (1 serving) = 630
- A taco salad (1 serving) = 900
- Cobb salad with grilled chicken (1 serving) = 1130
- Oriental grilled chicken salad (1 serving) = 1290
- A chili quesadilla salad (1 serving) = 1430

Calories from Meat, Poultry, and Fish			
1 Double cheeseburger	440	Sirloin steak (grilled 4 ounces)	197
Lamb (broiled 4 ounces)	330	Veal (broiled 4 ounces)	192
Rib-eye-steak (grilled 4 ounces)	322	1 Hot dog (beef or pork)	188
1 Pork chop (broiled 4 ounces)	316	Salmon (cooked 4 ounces)	166
1 Hot dog with bun	272	Shrimp (cooked 4 ounces)	160
1 Hamburger patty (Ground beef 4 ounces)	250	Turkey breast (cooked boneless 4 ounces)	153
Battered fried fish (4 ounces)	226	Tuna (canned water 4 ounces)	132
Pork loin (broiled 4 ounces)	225	1 Chicken breast (boiled)	128
Chicken breast (grilled boneless 4 ounces)	200	Tilapia (cooked 4 ounces)	110

Calories from Other Common Foods			
Spaghetti Bolognese (regular serving)	1300	Egg salad bowl	260
Pasta Carbonara (regular serving)	1260	Mashed potatoes (1 cup)	227
Ravioli Bolognese (spinach ricotta)	650	Peanut butter (2 tablespoons)	180
Macaroni and cheese (regular serving)	376	Chicken veg. soup bowl (homemade)	162
Lasagna (with meat sauce- regular serving)	350	Ranch salad dressing (2 tablespoons)	146
Pizza (1 slice of pepperoni)	300	Bread (a slice of white wheat)	123
1 Bagel	290	Cheddar cheese (1 slice)	113
Spaghetti (1 cup cooked, no sauce)	287	Yogurt (low fat 100 gr.)	97
Chili with beans (1 cup)	287	Egg (one large hard-boiled)	77

Common Drinks (Calories)	
Coffee (1 cup Java Chip Frappuccino)	600
Beer (12 ounces regular)	150
Cola (12 ounces regular)	136
Milk (8 ounces 2%)	122
Beer (12 ounces light)	110
Wine (5 ounces red)	105
Orange juice (8 ounces from concentrate)	102
Wine (6 ounces white)	100
Coffee (1 cup regular black homemade)	2

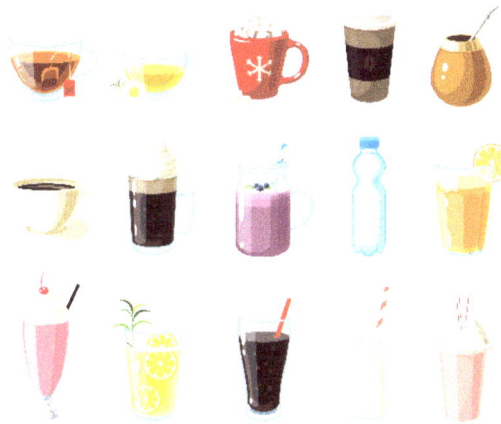

The number of calories we eat is one of the biggest contributing factors in gaining or losing weight. Regardless of our nutritional sources, the calories we ingest can be used as physical energy or stored in our bodies as fat. These extra calories will increase our weight unless we increase our activity to burn them.

Before filling our plates with food, remember that an average person needs to burn about 3500 calories of fat to lose one pound. Also, by cutting about 500 to 1,000 calories daily from our regular diet, we may lose about 1 to 2 pounds a week. According to the Mayo Clinic, the average calories for a healthy weight loss should be as follows:

Current Weight	Caloric Goals	
Pounds	Women	Men
250 or less	1,200	1,400
251 - 300	1,400	1,600
301 or more	1,600	1,800

Important Recommendation:

Become your own food expert and identify the eating habits that work and the ones that you need to modify to maintain a healthy weight. However, keep in mind that although all foods you eat contain calories, not all calories have the same effect on your overall health.

To keep in mind

- Carbohydrates should be eaten in their natural, whole, unprocessed form.

- Excessive fat intake is linked to chronic health disorders.

- Reducing food portions is one of the most effective ways to control your weight.

- Become aware of the caloric content in the foods you frequently eat.

Questions to reflect on:

1. Do you follow the 80/20 rule for healthy eating?

2. What are the main sources of natural sugars? Do you include them in your daily diet?

3. Why are complex carbohydrates healthier than simple ones? Do you include them in your regular diet?

4. Why are saturated and trans fats unhealthy? Do you usually avoid consuming them?

5. What types of foods make you gain the most weight? Are you aware of their caloric content?

Chapter 3:

Developing Healthier Eating and Drinking Habits

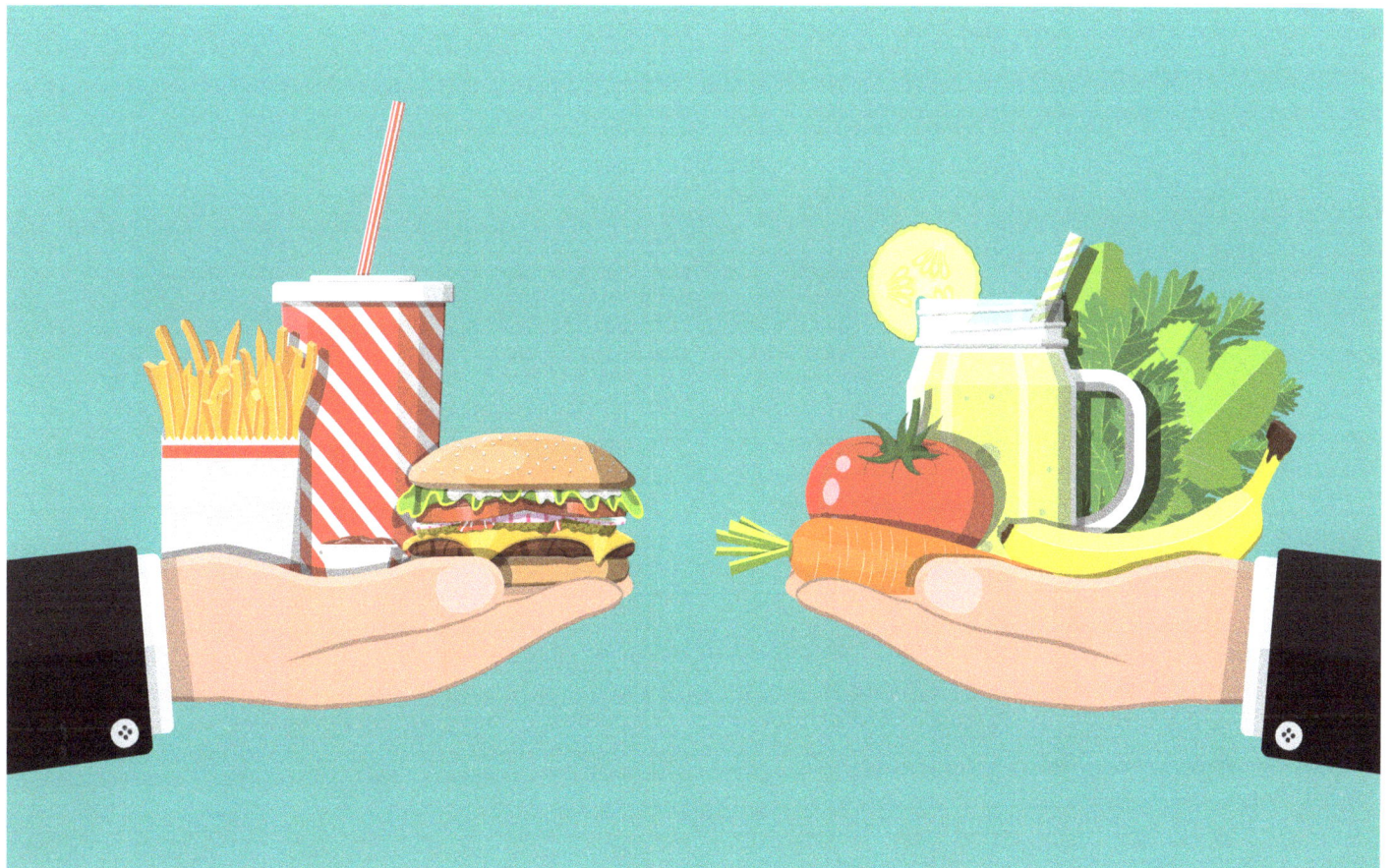

Many people consider eating one of life's greatest pleasures. Certainly, the anticipation of a tasty meal is appealing. Thus, food has always been a common denominator in many social activities and, on some occasions, even the focus of our lives. Feasts and celebrations include sharing elaborate meals with family and friends. However, the excessive emphasis on food intake in modern society has become a serious problem for most people.

The process of adopting smart eating habits usually begins at home. But even when parents promote good nutritional practices, relatives or friends may unintentionally undermine their efforts. Some of us do not recognize the terrible disservice to children every time we reward them with sweet and salty treats. We cause their taste buds to develop a preference or even become addicted to unhealthy foods. Parents and adults are responsible for teaching children to make healthy food choices.

Because fast foods are available everywhere, being mindful of our eating habits is crucial to a healthy lifestyle. It is often said that we are what we eat and drink. Ironically, many eat meals while distracted by our phones, computers, or televisions. These distractions prevent us from enjoying food and being aware of what and how we eat. However, to develop a healthy relationship with food, we must consider what, when, where, and why we eat.

To determine if your environment promotes healthy eating, consider answering these questions:

- Are you surrounded by food or by people who are compulsive eaters at home, school, or work?

- Do you plan your meals or eat whatever is available whenever you feel hungry?

- Do you favor certain foods, regardless of their nutritional value or simply because they taste better than others?

- Do you frequently eat out, order food, or cook pre-made frozen meals?

- Do you allow others to determine what ingredients go into your food and mouth?

Eating mindfully entails paying attention to our eating habits and changing food routines that prevent us from maintaining a healthy weight. Most people can successfully make lasting improvements in their lives because, in more instances, their bodies can adapt to changes that they consciously introduce.

It may not always be easy, but when we begin adopting healthy nutritional practices, we are more likely to make other positive changes to increase our overall wellness. Here are some key nutritional strategies that have helped me age well and maintain good health.

1. Eating slowly and mindfully. This is the most important reason for me to maintain a slim figure well into my golden years. I am totally convinced that eating slowly is crucial for good health and weight control. I always force myself to eat slowly because I recognize that good eating habits begin with chewing carefully for proper digestion. I believe anyone can benefit from eating slowly and enjoying every bite of their food.

Whether I eat by myself or with others, I cut my food into small pieces, chew them carefully, and swallow them before taking the next bite. I also set my silverware down between bites and pause to sip my beverage. As a result, I always feel satisfied way before I finish my meal. That is when I stop eating.

According to research, people who eat slowly and mindfully have leaner bodies because they feel full sooner and eat less food. Eating slowly gives our digestive system sufficient time to tell our brain that we are full. This process normally takes about 20 minutes. Furthermore, eating slowly allows us plenty of time to savor a meal and enjoy the eating experience even more.

2. Controlling portion sizes. Portion sizes have been getting larger in our homes and restaurants, which compels people to overeat. In addition, food makers are packaging their products in larger sizes. In a way, we have been forced to treat our bodies like food processors, loading them with unnecessary calories.

Given that we usually tend to overindulge when faced with super-size portions, we must learn to exert moderation as we eat in or out. Learning to serve the right-sized portions helps us prevent excessive calorie intake and unwanted weight gain.

To start, using smaller plates and glasses is a good idea. They make food and drink servings look bigger. The bigger the plate, the bigger the meal, and the bigger the person. In contrast, the less we eat, the less we need to satisfy our hunger. Soon, this change will translate into a smaller waistline.

I also recommend bringing food to the table in individual plates, instead of passing the serving dishes around. This smart and healthy way of eating has always been customary in my family, and I can attest to its good results in preventing anyone from getting seconds or extra helpings we do not need. We manage to program ourselves to eat only what we have in front of us to feel satisfied.

People do not need to measure portions or weigh food every time they eat, but filling half the plate with vegetables or a mixture of vegetables and fruits is highly recommended. The rest of the plate should have some lean protein and a side. It also helps to become portion savvy and learn what constitutes adequate meal portions for common foods. For example:

- Breakfast cereal= 30g or three tablespoons
- Lean meat or chicken = 100g or a portion the size of a deck of cards
- Fish= 150g
- Pizza= 1 medium slice
- Rice= one cup (6 tablespoons)
- Pasta= one cup (6 tablespoons)
- A small baked potato
- Vegetables= 85g

Additional recommendations for portion control include:

- **Eating your meals at regular times** (the hungrier you get, the more you tend to eat.)

- **Getting accustomed to eating until you are satisfied** and not waiting until you feel full.

- **Drinking a full glass of water before sitting to eat a meal** (Water starts to fill you up and prevents overeating.) It works!

3. Preparing your food and eating most of your meals at home. Our hectic way of life has made restaurant and pre-packaged meals very convenient for us. However, we do not realize that the less we cook, the more weight we tend to gain.

Eating out is associated with more empty calories, less nutritional value, and, sometimes, more alcohol consumption. In contrast, home cooking favors healthy eating because the meals that most of us prepare usually contain less salt, fat, sugar, and additives.

Eating out or getting take-out food may be a quick solution when someone is in a hurry. However, preparing healthy foods requires little time or advanced cooking skills. It only takes a little planning, creativity, and willingness to cook. Moreover, the most nutritious meals are the ones in which the ingredients remain close to their original fresh form.

Additional recommendations for food preparation:

- **If you need more basic cooking skills,** consider taking a few lessons to learn some cooking principles and encourage yourself to prepare your dishes. Once you start cooking regularly, you will become more creative in mixing ingredients according to your taste. You can also put together a collection of healthy recipes you enjoy preparing. In addition, you can find new appliances and utensils to simplify the home cooking process.

- **Keep spices, dried herbs, and garlic in your pantry to prepare fast-healthy meals.** Also, have tuna, canned sardines, high-bran crackers, brown rice, whole-wheat pasta, lentils, oatmeal, or any other ingredient that you can use regularly. Have fresh or frozen fruits and vegetables, eggs, turkey, and various low-fat cheeses in your fridge.

- **Avoid buying chips, fried foods, cookies, cakes, ice cream, or sugary drinks.** However, if you still decide to do it, keep them out of sight in a high cabinet or in the back of the freezer. Chances are, you will forget you have them but will only have access to them when an occasional craving arises.

- **Many supermarkets offer an excellent variety of fresh ingredients that can be used in simple recipes** that might take less than 30 minutes to cook. Also, a large selection of healthy recipes is available online, in books, and in magazines. Keep in mind that the more frequently you prepare a dish, the easier it becomes.

- **To save time,** you can cook in bulk two or three dishes a week and store them in portion-sized containers to be conveniently heated or eaten.

- **Place fresh vegetables and fruits at the center of your nutrition** because they are delicious, nutritious, and easy to fix and digest. Vegetables can be combined into salads or added to different types of soups.

- **Cooking soups with fish,** seafood, chicken, or turkey simplifies life and provides quick, satisfying meals. Broth-based homemade soups that contain protein are as filling as solid foods; therefore, they can be served as an entire meal and provide many healthy nutrients.

- **Try to plan some of your weekly meals and make a shopping list to speed up the grocery-buying process.** When you get home, cut fruits and vegetables and portion them in containers so that they are ready to be used in a meal.

- **Various companies offer fresh products in convenient packages, ready to be fixed.** The recipes are also included. This service gives you more control over ingredients and portion sizes, although it might be pricier. However, it is still much healthier and cheaper than eating out.

- **Bring your own lunch to work as often as possible**. When people are exposed to various appealing food alternatives while they wait in line in a cafeteria, they feel less inclined to control what they eat.

- **Eat out only on special occasions and consider it an enjoyable activity**. If you tend to eat more at a restaurant, try to take half of your meal home. In addition, if you know you will have a splurge meal, reduce the amount of food you consume before and after eating out.

4. Eating 30 to 40 grams of fiber daily. Dietary fiber is a food component needed for a healthy digestive system, although it is not digested or absorbed by the body. It facilitates food metabolism and keeps the digestive tract functioning optimally. A high-fiber diet is associated with good health and longevity.

Fiber comes in two forms: soluble and insoluble. Soluble fiber dissolves in water and is absorbed into the bloodstream. It turns into a gel in the stomach and slows digestion. Therefore, it helps lower and regulate blood sugar and cholesterol levels. Insoluble fiber remains in the digestive system and keeps food moving in the intestinal tract, facilitating the digestive process.

Eating more plant foods such as vegetables, fruits, nuts, seeds, whole grains, and beans is the best way to get enough fiber in your diet. The average person only gets 15 grams of fiber daily. You should aim to get between 30 to 40 grams of fiber from various foods and supplements. To increase fiber consumption, replace refined carbs such as white flour, white bread, white pasta, and white rice with whole-grain items.

A high-fiber diet has many benefits for your health:

- It normalizes bowel movements and maintains bowel health. It prevents constipation and lowers your risk of colon cancer.

- It lowers blood pressure, inflammation, and cholesterol levels. It reduces the risk of cardiovascular disease and most cancers.

- It lowers the risk of developing type 2 diabetes.

- It promotes weight loss. People who eat whole-grain foods tend to be thinner because they are likely to eat less and stay satisfied longer.

Here is a list of high-fiber foods:

Fruits	Vegetables	Grains and beans	Nuts and seeds
apples	avocado	brown and wild rice	almonds
bananas	broccoli	oats	peanuts
blackberries	carrots	whole wheat	pecans
blueberries	corn	barley	hazelnuts
kiwis	cabbage	quinoa	walnuts
mangos	kale	rye	cashews
oranges	lettuce	beans	chia seeds
peaches	spinach	green beans	flax seeds
pineapple	tomatoes	lentils	sunflower seeds
strawberries	zucchini	peas	pumpkin seeds

5. Reducing salt intake and avoiding high-salt foods. It is well-known that while salt is a necessary nutrient for good health, too much salt is unhealthy. The problem with diets high in sodium is that they are linked to many chronic conditions, such as high blood pressure, heart disease, stroke, and kidney failure.

Salt increases blood volume, which makes the heart work harder and raises blood pressure. High blood pressure damages blood vessels and arteries, provoking strokes and heart attacks. Salt also causes fluid retention and promotes weight gain by increasing fat consumption.

Most foods and drinks contain hidden amounts of sodium. Packaged, processed and restaurant foods have even higher amounts because salt is the most common flavoring ingredient food makers use. Although many foods do not taste salty, they may still contain sodium, such as cheese and bread, for instance.

Health organizations recommend that an average healthy adult consumes between 1.5 and 2.3 grams of salt daily, which is between 1 and 1 ½ teaspoons a day. They advise reducing sodium intake using fresh rather than cured, smoked, and packaged meats.

Fresh cuts of beef, chicken, or pork contain natural sodium, but their content is lower than the extra sodium added during processing in products like bacon, ham, or sausages. If a food item keeps well in the fridge for several days or weeks, it is a sign that its sodium content is too high.

Salt preference is an acquired food habit. Therefore, it can be modified by gradually reducing the amount of salt that you use in your meals. It takes about six weeks for your taste buds to get used to eating less salt, but once they do, you will learn to dislike salty foods.

Tips to reduce salt usage:

- Use garlic, salt-free seasonings, and spices, herbs, or lemon juice to enhance food flavors.

- Add less salt than what a recipe calls for.

- Avoid buying packaged and canned foods unless labeled "Low-sodium" or "No salt added."

- Read food labels to detect salt content and pay attention to serving sizes.

- Limit the use of sauces, mixes, and instant products.

- Keep takeout and fast foods as an occasional treat

- Break the habit of reaching out for your saltshaker by keeping it away from your table.

6. Reducing sugar intake and artificial sweeteners. Natural sugar, which is present in fruits, vegetables, grains, and dairy is recommended because these items offer a regular supply of energy to our cells. In contrast, health authorities warn that added sugars are toxic, addictive, and quite destructive to our bodies.

They promote the development of chronic diseases and speed up the aging process resulting in sagging skin and wrinkles.

Our modern diet is rich in processed sugars and artificial sweeteners. Thus, the average person consumes about 160 grams of fructose a day (or 38 teaspoons.) However, the daily recommendation is only about 30 grams (or seven teaspoons.)

Refined sugars added to sodas, juices, cereals, candy, pastries, desserts, and so on produce significant weight gain, raising the risk of obesity and diabetes. They are also responsible for inflammation, heart disease, and some cancers.

High daily consumption of sugar puts a lot of pressure on the liver to metabolize it and turns off its appetite-control system. It also stimulates the liver to produce fat cells, which are very difficult to eliminate. Usually, it takes about six days of sugar excess to cause insulin resistance and to disrupt someone's hormonal balance.

Recommendations to reduce sugar intake:

- Read food labels for information on the amount of sugar added per serving so that you can keep track of your sugar intake and make better food choices. The most common sugars are sucrose, glucose, lactose, and fructose. Keep in mind that fruit juices, beverages, and cocktails are loaded with sugar.

- Cut back on sugar consumption to maintain a healthy weight and prevent degenerative illnesses. Learn to curb your sweet tooth habit and control your sugar cravings because the more sugar you consume, the more you will need to satisfy your sweet impulses. The opposite is also true. As you gradually reduce dietary sugars, your taste buds will adjust to a low-sugar diet.

Overcoming a sugar dependency or addiction is challenging for anyone, but it has many benefits. You will protect brain cells from damage and keep a sharp mind. You will maintain stable and brighter moods as well as long-lasting energy. You will be able to reduce visceral fat, look younger and live longer. These positive effects will soon be reflected in your overall health and wellness.

7. Limiting alcohol consumption. Although alcohol is present in various social interactions, parties, and meals, its impact on our health is extensively debated in the medical field. For instance, nutritionists believe that alcohol is not an essential nutrient; therefore, it is not a required item in our regular diet. Thus, not drinking it does not lead to any nutritional deficiency.

Medical studies either support a moderate consumption of alcohol or warn against its negative impact on our health. Some physicians state that drinking an occasional glass of red wine or a beer may contribute to good health and could even be associated with longevity.

In contrast, detractors of alcohol claim that its toxicity outweighs the few benefits it may have. In their opinion, alcohol is a drug that impairs a person's performance, may cause addiction, damages our organs, and is associated with most auto accident fatalities.

To determine if we want to drink alcohol occasionally or avoid it altogether, we need to understand how it affects the human body. Alcoholic beverages, regardless of their origin, contain three main ingredients: water, ethanol, and various amounts of sugar. The alcoholic content of a drink depends on the technique used to make it.

One of the many problems with alcohol consumption is that humans lack the ability to process and store it. We also lack the mechanism that prevents us from feeling satisfied by alcoholic drinks. Therefore, drinking to excess and the potential of becoming addicted to alcohol can cause serious problems for anyone.

Once alcohol enters our system, our liver makes it a priority to metabolizing it. It intends to prevent alcohol from harming our cells and organs. As a result, the drink goes into our bloodstream immediately and raises our blood alcohol concentration (BAC) quite rapidly. Its effects reach our brains within minutes.

Although each individual processes alcohol a little differently, the average person metabolizes between 7 to 14 grams of alcohol per hour, which is equivalent to one beer or half a drink. Alcohol should be consumed slowly (preferably alternating it with water) to give your liver enough time to metabolize it.

It is imperative to remember that regular alcohol consumption adds calories to our diet, and it contributes to weight gain and abdominal obesity. Normally, a gram of alcohol contains about seven calories, while mixed drinks and cocktails have many more. It is easy for us to drink calories at a fast pace.

The following table provides information on the caloric content of some common alcoholic drinks.

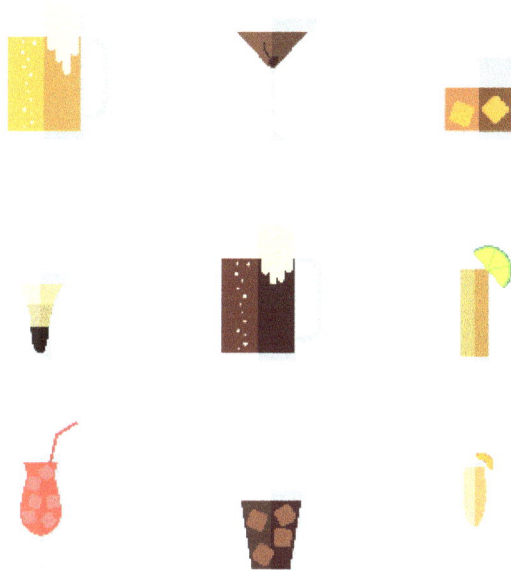

Caloric Content for Common Alcoholic Drinks	
Mai tai 4 oz	310
Martini 4 oz	276
Margarita 4 oz	270
Pina colada 4.5 oz	245
Mojito cocktail 4 oz	217
Frozen daiquiri 4 oz	216
White or red wine (sweet) 5 oz	180
Regular beer 12 oz	150
Champagne or sparkling wine 5 oz	125
Gin 1.5 oz	110
Red wine 5 oz	105
Whiskey 1.5 oz	105
White wine (dry) 5 oz	100
Vodka 1.5 oz	96
Rum 1.5 oz	96
Tequila 1.5 oz	96

Recommendations for alcohol consumption:

- Think twice before having or ordering another drink because alcohol intake increases a person's appetite and food intake. If you are trying to lose or maintain a healthy weight, avoid alcohol as much as possible.

- To reduce or control your alcohol intake, learn to drink slowly, and make your drink last longer. Eat something before you have an alcoholic drink and accompany it with regular or sparkling water.

- Whenever you choose to consume alcohol, do it responsibly. That is, know how much alcohol you can drink safely without putting yourself or anyone in danger. Be kind to your liver, yourself, and others. Consider that alcohol impairs your thinking and reflexes. Therefore, you should never drink and drive.

8. Adopting a Mediterranean style of eating. The Mediterranean diet is plant-based and more than a conventional restrictive food plan. It is based on foods available in Southern Italy and Greece, and it has been recommended by the World Health Organization and the American Dietary Guidelines as an ideal eating diet.

The Mediterranean way of eating is believed to be responsible for the good health and longevity of the people in these two Southern European regions. These places have the highest percentage of over 90 years of age, and they have more centenarians per capita than the United States. The Mediterranean way of life also includes being physically active and enjoying relaxing meals with other people.

Although there are different variations of this diet, the following pyramid illustrates the various products that are included.

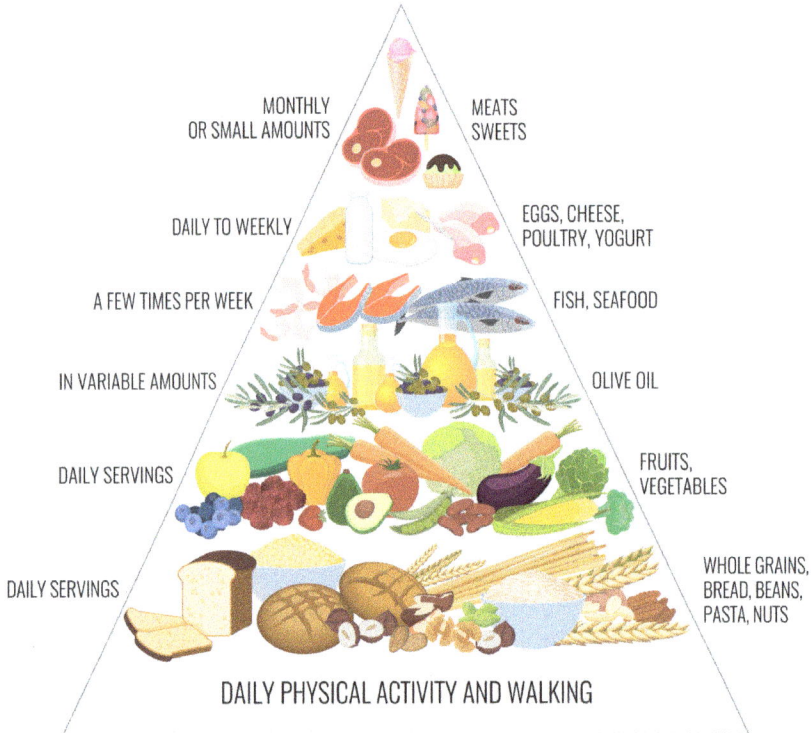

MONTHLY OR SMALL AMOUNTS — MEATS SWEETS

DAILY TO WEEKLY — EGGS, CHEESE, POULTRY, YOGURT

A FEW TIMES PER WEEK — FISH, SEAFOOD

IN VARIABLE AMOUNTS — OLIVE OIL

DAILY SERVINGS — FRUITS, VEGETABLES

DAILY SERVINGS — WHOLE GRAINS, BREAD, BEANS, PASTA, NUTS

DAILY PHYSICAL ACTIVITY AND WALKING

MEDITERRANEAN DIET

The Mediterranean diet emphasizes consuming lots of fruits, vegetables, whole grains, nuts, and seeds. It also includes eating healthy plant-based fats like olive oil and avocados or fish like salmon and sardines. (Olive oil is considered liquid gold for cardiovascular care.) Fish and seafood are the main sources of animal proteins, while other animal proteins like poultry are eaten less frequently and in smaller portions.

Overall, red meat is consumed only about three times a month on average. Water is the preferred drink, although a moderate intake of wine is accepted. In short, according to this diet, we should have a:

- **Daily** consumption of **olive oil**, **fruits** and **vegetables**, **legumes,** and **whole grains**
- **Weekly** consumption of **fish**, **seafood**, **poultry,** and **eggs**
- **Moderate** consumption of **dairy products** (milk, cheese, yogurt)
- **Moderate** consumption of **wine** or **beer** (preferably red wine)
- **Low** consumption of **red meat**, **natural fats,** and **desserts**

Several studies have shown that the Mediterranean diet increases life expectancy and reduces premature death. It offers significant health benefits such as:

- Preventing heart disease and strokes by reducing risk factors such as high blood pressure, triglycerides, and cholesterol.
- Protecting against type 2 diabetes and promoting healthy weight management by stabilizing blood sugar levels.
- Boosting brain health and memory by decreasing the risk of cognitive decline, dementia, Alzheimer's, and Parkinson's diseases.
- Strengthening bones by preserving bone density and preventing osteoporosis.
- Reducing the incidence of cancer, especially breast and colon cancer.
- Lowering the risk of depression.

I support and follow this nutritional diet because it happens to be a delicious way to help my body age well and prevent many diseases. Furthermore, it is inexpensive, balanced, and quite satisfying.

My typical breakfast, for instance, is a mixture of oats, chia, flax seeds, nuts, plain yogurt, and at least three different fresh fruits like bananas, blueberries, and strawberries. It gives me enough energy in the morning, and it helps me maintain stable sugar levels until lunch.

You can find many Mediterranean recipes on the internet. Here is a suggested week's menu to get you started.

Monday:
Breakfast: Greek yogurt with strawberries and oats.
Lunch: A sandwich **of whole grain bread** with vegetables.
Dinner: A tuna salad dressed in olive oil and fruit for dessert.

Tuesday:
Breakfast: Oatmeal with milk and raisins.
Lunch: Chicken soup with vegetables.
Dinner: Salad with tomatoes, olives, and feta cheese.

Wednesday:
Breakfast: Omelet with veggies, tomatoes, and onions. A piece of fruit.
Lunch: A sandwich on whole grain bread with cheese and fresh vegetables.
Dinner: Mediterranean lasagna.

Thursday:
Breakfast: Greek yogurt with strawberries and oats.
Lunch: A sandwich with vegetables **on whole grain bread**.
Dinner: A tuna salad dressed in olive oil. A piece of fruit for dessert.

Friday:
Breakfast: Greek yogurt with strawberries and oats.
Lunch: A whole grain bread sandwich with vegetables.
Dinner: A tuna salad dressed in olive oil. A piece of fruit for dessert.

Saturday:
Breakfast: Oatmeal with raisins, nuts, and an apple.
Lunch: Whole grain bread sandwich with vegetables.
Dinner: Mediterranean pizza made with whole wheat, topped with cheese, vegetables and olives.

Sunday:
Breakfast: Omelet with veggies and olives.
Lunch: Leftover pizza from the night before.
Dinner: Grilled chicken with vegetables and a potato. Fruit for dessert.

(source: www.healthline.com) https://www.healthline.com/nutrition/mediterranean-diet-meal-plan#sample-menu

Note: that the Mediterranean diet does not require specific portion sizes or calorie counting; therefore, you can determine the portion size that satisfies your hunger.

9. Practicing intermittent fasting. Although fasting is a current fitness trend, it has been a universal, ancient religious practice. It refers to the voluntary restriction or abstinence from foods or drinks for a certain period of time. Fasting is supported by experts in the medical field worldwide. It is associated with great benefits for the body and the brain and for contributing to longevity.

It is well-accepted that humans can function without food for days and even weeks. Once a person begins fasting, the body gets the energy needed from the glucose stored in the liver and muscles. This process starts about 8 hours after the last meal.

Once the glucose reserves have been depleted, the body begins burning fat to produce energy. It needs to be emphasized that the body does not use muscle to produce energy until all fat stored in the body has been used. Using fat for energy preserves muscle mass and reduces cholesterol.

Fasting is the most effective way to balance insulin levels because almost all foods raise blood sugar. Therefore, regular fasting reduces insulin resistance in a significant way. Even though hunger is mainly a temporary effect of fasting, our appetite gradually decreases as our body adjusts to intermittent fasting. A few days after fasting, people often experience higher levels of endorphins, increasing mental well-being and feeling more energetic.

There are various types of fasting:

Intermittent fasting: refers to alternating days in which food intake is reduced or totally restricted with regular eating days.

The 16-8 fasting: abstaining from eating for 16 hours a day followed by an 8-hour eating period. For example, if your last meal is at 6:00 pm, your breakfast the next day should be at 10:00 am on a fasting day.

Calorie restriction fasting: implies reducing calorie intake to the minimum in fasting days (usually twice a week) to about 500 calories for women and 600 for men.

Partial fasting: requires eliminating certain foods or drinks during fasting periods.

Water or juice fasting: involves drinking only water, fruit, or vegetable juices on fasting days.

Notice that fasting is not a diet but an eating pattern that restricts food intake. Fasting is not recommended for children, pregnant women, or people who are underweight or who have a history of eating disorders or health problems. Although fasting is beneficial to most people, it is advisable to consult with your doctor beforehand.

Fasting will be most beneficial when combined with a well-balanced diet rich in vegetables, fruits, lean proteins, and healthy fats, to compensate for any lack of nutrients associated with this food reduction. It is also important to be properly hydrated while fasting. By reducing the overall calorie intake, all fasting modalities should cause weight loss. That is, provided that you don't overeat during the alternating eating periods.

To keep in mind

- Eating mindfully means paying attention to your eating habits and food routines to maintain a healthy weight.

- Prepare your own food because eating out usually makes people gain weight.

- Control sugar cravings, reduce salt intake and limit alcohol consumption for better health.

- Adopt a Mediterranean style of eating based on fruits, vegetables, whole grains, nuts, and seeds.

Questions to reflect on:

1. What are some of the benefits of eating slowly? Can you adopt this healthy habit?

2. What recommendations for food portion control can you follow?

3. Why is eating out or buying take-out less healthy than cooking your own meals? Is eating out frequently a contributing factor to your weight gain?

4. What healthy eating habits might most benefit you?

Chapter 4:

Obesity and Managing Weight Loss

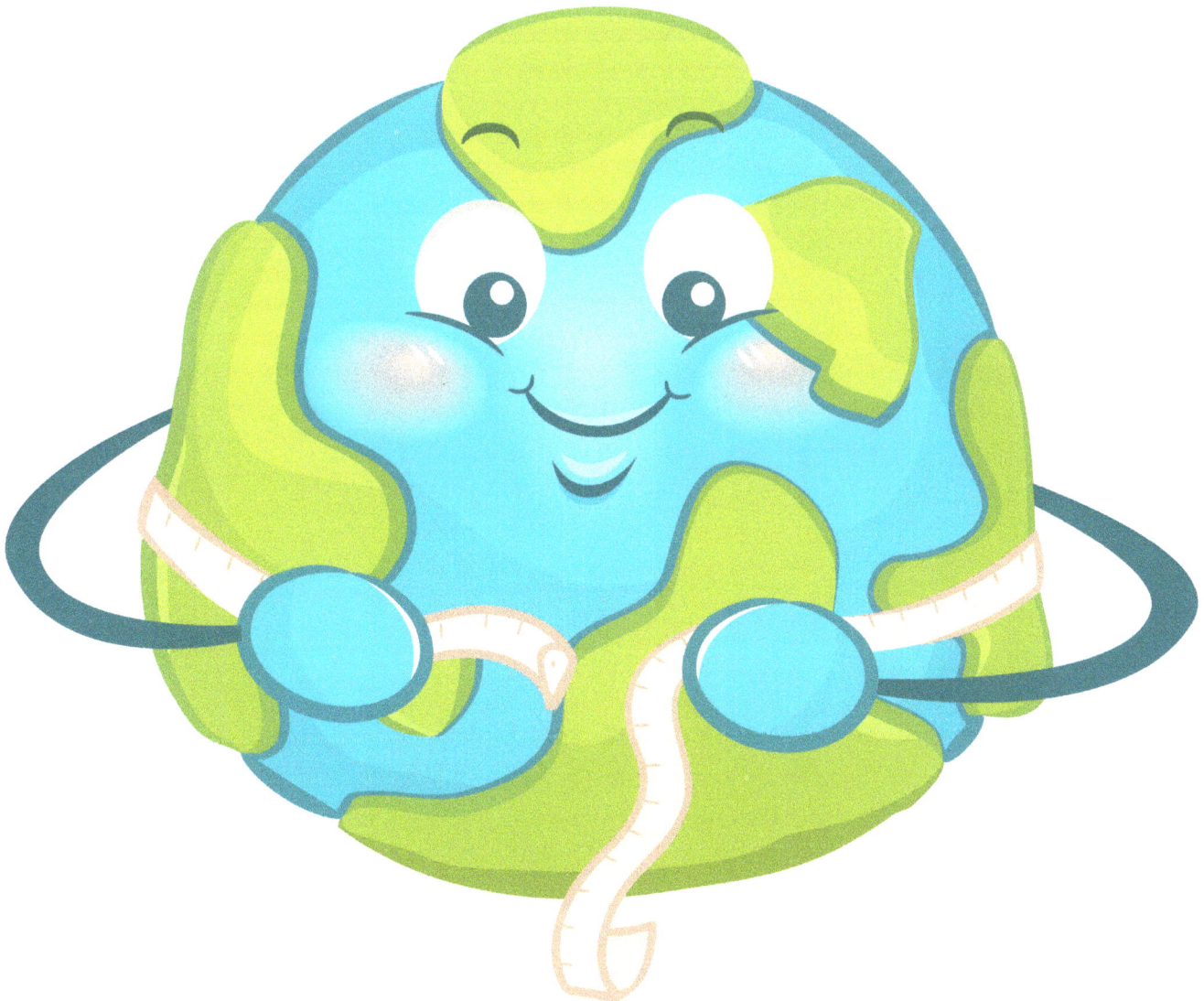

All over the world, obesity, which has been rare in most of human history, has become an epidemic since the 1970s. People everywhere are getting bigger and heavier to the point that being lean is becoming less and less common. Yet, although obesity rates keep growing at an alarming pace, affecting people in all age groups, we still seem somewhat oblivious to the gravity of this global crisis, which causes many health problems, unhappiness, and disability.

It seems ironic that in a short period, people have developed a keen sensibility and terror of the COVID-19 virus globally, while most of us keep disregarding the evident, devastating impact of obesity in our communities worldwide. But obesity is also a pandemic that requires urgent attention; it is considered a time bomb by medical researchers and physicians. For this reason, everyone must be aware of the nature of this preventable disease and the best ways to halt its growth. We must learn how to reduce the burden of obesity on our physical, emotional, and mental health.

The path to understanding and curing obesity has become difficult to navigate because it has been loaded with myths and one-sided approaches that often focus on specific culprits. Over the years, all of us have been exposed to confusing medical and nutritional information about the most effective treatments for this ailment. However, advanced research is finally unlocking the secrets of weight loss to remedy this modern disease.

Obesity is a chronic, progressive condition that begins when people gain small amounts of weight regularly. Before long, they are overweight or obese, and this pattern carries detrimental consequences for their overall well-being. Check the following body mass index (BMI) chart to be aware of your risk of developing obesity.

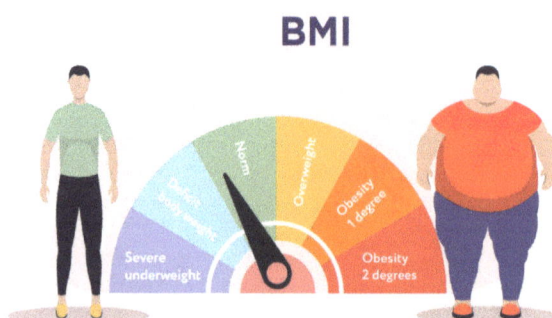

BMI

Body Mass Index Chart

Underweight: BMI is less than 18.5
Normal weight: BMI is 18.5 to 24.9
Overweight: BMI is 25 to 29.9
Obese: BMI is 30 or more

There are multiple driving factors of obesity, although damaging dietary practices and unhealthy lifestyle habits are the most recognized. The concrete underlying causes of obesity are not the same for every obese individual, as it happens with any other major illness. Becoming aware of the immediate and ultimate causes of our obesity will help us find the most effective treatment for this preventable disorder.

It can be said that the obesity crisis has been precipitated by the development of the convenience food industry, which has taken the responsibility of cooking away from us and our kitchens. As a result, we find it very convenient to buy or order precooked meals from fast food chains, restaurants, cafeterias, and supermarkets.

Unfortunately, many people ignore that most factory-made foods are loaded with artificial sweeteners, high salt, high fat, and various preservatives. They are also unaware that these extremely palatable foods can be highly addictive, they can ruin our taste buds, and alter our body and brain chemistry. Furthermore, they make us sluggish and obese.

Nutritionally polluted foods packed with anti-nutrients, hormones, and harmful chemicals can cause permanent damage to our organs, giving us heart disease, cancer, diabetes, depression, dementia, and other chronic disorders. In contrast, good quality food provides nutrition and sustenance, and it has a positive impact on our health. According to medical experts, most chronic illnesses can be improved with weight loss and a balanced diet without the typical cost and side effects of medication.

To prevent and cure obesity effectively, we must understand how our body metabolizes and stores energy and nutrients from the food we eat. We also need to learn about the impact of proper nourishment on our overall health and mental well-being, so that we can make appropriate nutritional choices for ourselves and our loved ones. Developing nutritional wisdom and a good relationship with food is our best tool to eradicate obesity.

Digestion and metabolism are the biochemical processes by which food and nutrients are broken down into smaller components to be assimilated into the body. In a simplified way, the small intestine absorbs most of the nutrients, and the circulatory system distributes them to other parts of the body. The bloodstream carries sugars, amino acids, and vitamins to the liver and muscles, where they are stored and used when needed. These important nutrients are required for energy, growth, and cell repair.

Understanding the role of hormones, such as insulin, in digestion and metabolism is also crucial to address the root causes of obesity. Insulin is the hormone that regulates the metabolism of carbohydrates, fats, and proteins by promoting the absorption of glucose from the bloodstream into the liver. Insulin helps balance blood glucose levels and tells the liver to store excess glucose and fat to be released when levels decrease.

In balanced insulin processing, the glucose levels generally go up after we eat while making the liver store fat and glucose to be used later. During fasting periods, insulin levels go down as we use our stored energy. If energy is retrieved from the liver, it deflates, and no fat is gained or lost. In addition, by alternating between high and low levels of insulin, the body does not build resistance. This process is illustrated in the following diagram created by Dr. Jason Fung in his book *The Obesity Code: Unlocking the Secrets of Weight Loss*:

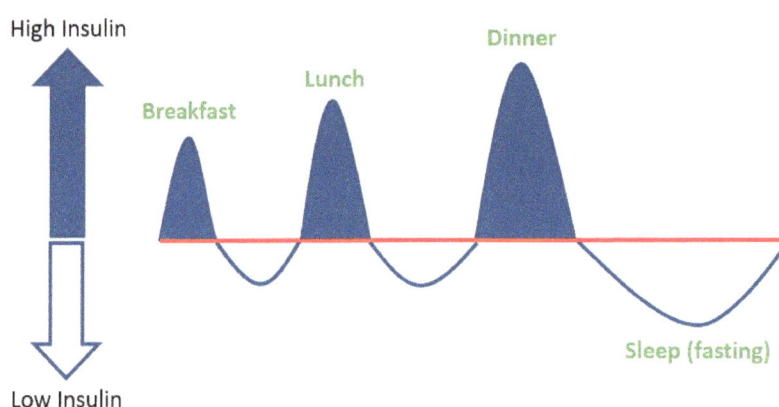

Insulin resistance, or impaired insulin sensitivity, happens when people develop tolerance to this hormone, thereby making it less effective. The pancreas is then forced to deploy higher amounts of insulin even though blood glucose levels continue to increase. But when the liver is already full of fat, higher insulin levels are needed to push more fat into the liver, causing insulin resistance. According to Dr. Fung, a leading expert in this anomaly, insulin resistance is the ultimate cause of both type 2 diabetes and obesity.

A diet high in sugars and other sources of refined carbohydrates, along with regular snacking, keeps insulin and glucose levels high. These foods lead to more glucose being available than needed, increasing fat storage. The excess fat and sugar are then accumulated as visceral fat (around the organs,) as subcutaneous fat (under the skin), and in the liver (leading to a fatty liver.)

Dr. Fung states that an imbalanced insulin processing may lead to resistance, which is illustrated below:

High Insulin

Dinner

Lunch

Breakfast

Snack   Snack   Snack

Sleep (fasting)

Low Insulin

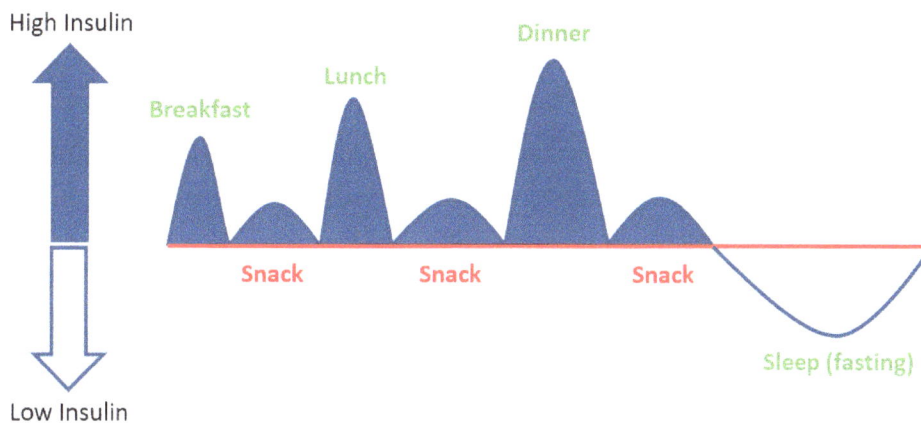

Insulin response is different between overweight and lean people. The former present a much higher tolerance to insulin; that is why obese people keep on gaining weight, even if they do not increase food intake significantly. Over time, obesity becomes both a hormonal and a caloric imbalance. The longer this cycle is maintained, the worse it becomes. In contrast, non-obese individuals have lower insulin levels, which reduce fat storage.

Insulin resistance affects the liver, the muscles, and the brain in different ways. An excess of insulin in the liver leads to liver insulin resistance. A sedentary lifestyle and minimal physical activity combined with high insulin levels promote muscle insulin resistance. When insulin resistance affects the brain, the body raises the body's set weight. Unfortunately, the longer a person carries extra weight, the more difficult it becomes to lose it and keep it off.

Another hormone associated with obesity is cortisol, also called the stress hormone. Cortisol makes glucose available to muscles during a temporary stressful situation, unlike insulin, which boosts glucose storage. It is essential to prepare the body for the short-term flight or fight response; however, under conditions of long-lasting or chronic stress, cortisol can elevate glucose levels leading to insulin release and eventually to insulin resistance.

Excess cortisol and stress cause weight gain and increase body mass index. Since sleep deprivation increases stress, it contributes to keeping cortisol and insulin levels high. The more sleep deprivation a person experiences, the higher the weight gain they have. These excesses promote abdominal obesity.

Abdominal fat accumulation is considered more dangerous to people's overall health than general weight gain, and it can be more difficult to eliminate. Too much visceral fat accumulation impairs organ function, increases inflammation, and raises the risk of chronic diseases. It is a sign of high cholesterol and heart disease. In addition, visceral fat releases hormones and toxins that damage the stomach, intestines, liver, and pancreas. A waistline higher than 35 inches for women and 40 inches for men indicates excess visceral fat.

Additional causes of obesity include binge eating and food addiction. Binge eating is an eating disorder characterized by an out-of-control urge to eat large amounts of food, followed by feelings of disgust and shame over that behavior. Food addiction happens when someone develops a chemical dependency on some foods, which makes eating them an extremely pleasurable experience. Long-compulsive overeating causes overstimulation of dopamine and changes in the brain reward system and often leads to obesity. These two compulsive disorders can be successfully treated with medical nutrition therapy.

There are important reasons why you must take weight gain and obesity seriously sooner rather than later:

You should not accept being overweight as a natural condition of your body, giving up on becoming healthier and fitter. Remember, your metabolism is a unique mechanism that maintains an optimal energy-spending balance so that you can have a leaner body. No one is genetically predisposed to overeat because nature has endowed us with hormones that warn us when we are full. Develop a healthy relationship with food and try to maintain a healthy weight. It is the most evident sign that you love yourself and that you are your own best friend.

Excess weight and obesity are associated with the main leading causes of death. They often prevent people from leading fulfilling, satisfying lives. The longer the risk factors are maintained, the bigger the damage to your health. The good news is that even a modest weight loss can produce significant health benefits at any age. By taking care of your own body, you are not only fulfilling your biggest responsibility but also helping to reduce healthcare costs for you, your family, and your government.

The sooner you adopt healthy habits, the higher your chances of keeping the weight off. Evidently, it is much easier to lose a few recently gained pounds than a large amount of extra weight carried over several years or decades. A high body set weight kept for a long time is more difficult to modify.

Excess body weight increases the risk of being discriminated against, bullied, or socially isolated. This situation severely impacts mental health leading to depression, low self-esteem, shame, and anxiety. By taking care of your body regularly, you can achieve a greater sense of happiness and well-being.

If you have been accumulating extra weight or are already obese, today is the right time to start managing your weight and turn things around. As the saying goes, there are two ideal moments to plant a tree: the first is a few years ago, and the second is today! There are no expiration dates on your ability to adopt healthy behaviors. Yet, the sooner you get rid of those excess pounds, the healthier you will be, the better you will look, and the most satisfied you will feel.

General Advice for Sustained Weight Loss

Many people believe that lasting weight loss is possible only when they find the most effective diet or when someone finally discovers a miracle drug that melts body fat. However, achieving a healthy weight is possible for everyone, including you.

The first step in your journey toward healthy weight management starts with identifying the behavioral, environmental, and emotional factors which have provoked your unwanted weight gain. Whether your issues involve inadequate nutritional choices, unhealthy eating patterns, bad lifestyle habits, or compulsive eating behaviors, these difficulties need to be addressed. That awareness will allow you to determine the most effective strategies for your long-term weight loss.

A diet program should not be something you do "on" and "off," but rather a healthy mindset that becomes part of your way of life. It should be made of principles and practices that guide your food selection, promote your regular physical activity, support your mental well-being, and help you maintain a fit and healthy body.

Scientific researchers have found evidence that small changes in lifestyle, whether it is adopting intermittent fasting, getting more sleep, reducing chronic stress, or increasing vigorous aerobic activity, can lead to permanent weight loss success. The following principles and tips can help you modify behaviors for weight loss:

1. Be mindful of your food intake and learn how to make the best nutritional choices.

Do more home cooking; it is vital to weight management and to leading a long healthy life. When you cook your meals, you are more aware of the ingredients, the proportions, and the freshness of your food. Good health starts in your kitchen, and cooking is the best thing you can do for yourself and your loved ones. Remember that ordering food and eating out frequently can become a health hazard.

Improve your eating habits; it is central to losing and maintaining your weight. To start, you need to burn more energy than you take in. That is the only way your weight will come off. To lose 1-2 pounds a week, you need to reduce your food intake by at least 500 calories a day and increase movement.

Eat real, fresh, unprocessed, chemical-free, whole foods as much as possible to energize you and keep you satisfied. Avoid refined, processed foods that are rich in sugars, salt, starchy carbs, unhealthy fats, and chemical additives; they contain a lot of calories but lack the essential components for balanced nutrition.

Increase vegetable and animal protein intake to promote satiety, boost metabolism, and maintain muscle mass while losing weight. Avoid processed meats, but eat lean, fresh, grass-fed meat. Get your proteins from food sources, not from supplements.

Add at least 30 grams of dietary fiber to your meals daily. Fiber is a great aid in weight loss because it reduces hunger, increases satiety, decreases caloric intake, and lowers caloric absorption. It also reduces insulin, glucose, and cholesterol levels. Almost all plant foods in their natural state contain fiber. Supplements can be helpful, too.

Drink 1-2 teaspoons of diluted apple cider to help you lose weight. It is a health tonic that reduces fat storage, improves metabolism, and prevents insulin resistance.

Eat and drink probiotic-rich foods and beverages for gut health and optimal digestion. Fermented foods like traditional pickles, sauerkraut, kefir, and yogurt with live and active cultures increase energy levels, control junk food cravings, reduce belly fat, and favor healthy weight management.

Modify your drinking habits by increasing water and unsweetened green tea consumption (infused with sliced lemons and oranges). To optimize weight loss, reduce alcohol, especially liquor and cocktails, and stay away from sweetened beverages and fruit juices. They all raise insulin levels and increase your appetite, leading you to eat more.

Restructure environments that promote overeating and excessive food availability. Also, keep an eye on hectic work schedules, worksite dining facilities, and vending machines because they contribute to the development of undesirable eating patterns.

Become aware of the way you interact with food to prevent emotional eating. Feelings such as boredom, stress, anger, sadness, tiredness, etc., may lead you to use food as a way of coping with these emotions. Also, identify the factors that increase your food cravings. Drink water and distract your mind from beating cravings.

Avoid strict, restrictive diets that make you feel hungry or unsatisfied. Losing weight through deprivation or suffering is the wrong strategy for maintaining a long-term commitment.

Consider adopting the Mediterranean diet as a balanced nutritional approach that promotes longevity and contributes to maintaining a healthy weight. In addition, combine it with gradual intermittent fasting to boost your body's metabolic engine.

Note: for additional information on healthy nutrition habits, consult the section: Understanding Key Nutritional Concepts and Calorie Intake, in this book.

2. Reduce sitting time and become more physically active. Exercise is vital in reaching and maintaining a healthy weight. Vigorous activity is the optimal complement to a healthy diet.

Create an energy management plan to get your body out of fat storage into a fat-burning mood. To start losing weight, you need at least 30 minutes of aerobic exercise 5 times a week.

If you have not exercised in a long time, increase energy expenditure gradually until you develop a sustainable movement plan. Begin with small steps to challenge yourself to move more often, like taking short walks in your neighborhood.

If you are moderately active, increase the amount of time you spend exercising. Design a routine you can stick with and explore alternative activities you may enjoy doing or consider worthy of your best efforts.

Note: for additional information on exercise, consult the section *Understanding the Effects of Exercise on Wellness* in this book.

3. Find a powerful source of motivation and support to drive you towards your goals. It will help you build inner strength and be prepared to overcome obstacles. Perhaps, you need to think about the reasons why you must lose weight and stay healthy.

4. Make yourself accountable and monitor your progress on a regular basis to prevent procrastination. People are naturally encouraged by improvements, and even small wins impact the motivational energy centers in your brain. On the other hand, you will not be able to control your weight without taking control of your actions.

5. Weigh yourself regularly, but do not worry about your weight. Use that information to measure your progress, reassess your goals, reinforce your determination to shed pounds off, and prevent you from regaining the weight you have already lost. Use the following chart as a reference:

Ideal Weight Chart		
Height	Women	Men
5´0´´	90 – 110 lbs	95 – 117 lbs
5´1´´	95 – 116 lbs	101 – 123 lbs
5´2´´	99 – 121 lbs	106 – 130 lbs
5´3´´	104 – 127 lbs	112 – 136 lbs
5´4´´	108 – 132 lbs	117 – 143 lbs
5´5´´	113 – 138 lbs	122 – 150 lbs
5´6´´	117 – 143 lbs	128 – 156 lbs
5´7´´	122 – 149 lbs	133 – 166 lbs
5´8´´	126 – 154 lbs	139 – 169 lbs
5´9´´	131 – 160 lbs	144 – 176 lbs
5´10´´	135 – 165 lbs	179 – 183 lbs
5´11´´	140 – 171 lbs	155 – 189 lbs
6´0´´	144 – 176 lbs	160 – 196 lbs
6´1´´	149 – 182 lbs	166 – 202 lbs
6´2´´	153 – 187 lbs	171 – 209 lbs

6. A steady weight loss of 1-2 pounds per week is the most doable and effective long-term weight management option. Accelerated weight loss plans are neither healthy nor sustainable, and they often lead to frustrating weight regain. People who have overcome obesity and have kept their weight off a long-term report that their secret includes a slow but steady weight loss, keeping track of their food intake, and increasing their physical activity levels.

Changing your old habits is a difficult task, but it can be done successfully with a realistic plan, commitment, and patience. The are no miracles involved in losing weight and improving your health; only a positive attitude and a great deal of determination will help you achieve your goals.

To keep in mind

- Obesity is a chronic, progressive condition that begins when people gain small amounts of weight regularly.

- You should not accept being overweight as a natural condition of your body, giving up on becoming healthier and fitter.

- Developing nutritional wisdom and a good relationship with food is the best tool to eradicate obesity.

- Excess weight and obesity are associated with the main leading causes of death.

Questions to reflect on:

1. Are you very concerned about your weight gain or that of a loved one? Explain

2. What role does insulin play in the digestion and metabolism process?

3. Why should you avoid developing insulin resistance?

4. What is the impact of abdominal fat accumulation on people's overall health?

5. Identify two main actions you intend to do to prevent or control obesity?

Chapter 5:

Effects of Exercise on Well-Being

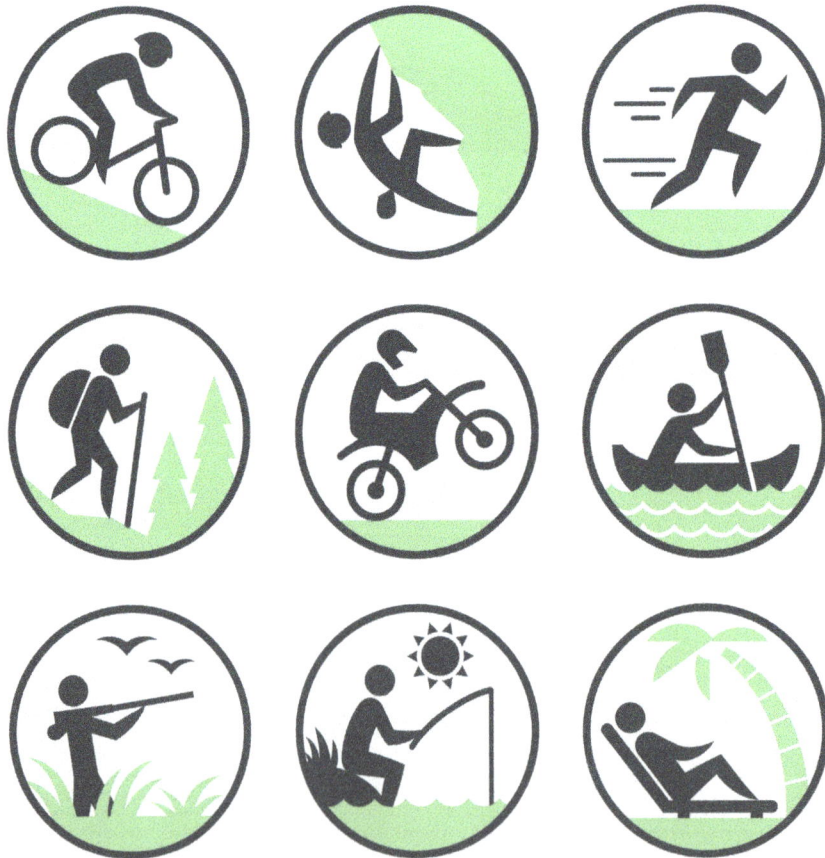

It is worth repeating that having a well-balanced diet and incorporating regular exercise in our daily lives are the two most important factors in protecting our physical and mental health. They also help us overcome the challenges of aging. Regular physical activity is a very effective way to reduce health deterioration. According to experts, there is no way around it: everyone needs to exercise regularly to live better and longer.

School, work, and modern lifestyles are becoming very sedentary, involving occupational and leisure sitting for long hours. Unfortunately, prolonged sitting and a sedentary lifestyle are the leading causes of premature death. These behaviors increase the risk of cardiovascular diseases, diabetes, and obesity. In contrast, current scientific studies provide compelling evidence that vigorous exercise is the antidote to these and many other ailments.

According to the Physical Activity Guidelines for Americans, about 80% of adults and adolescents in the U.S. do not meet the exercise requirements to maintain a healthy body, even though it is well known that exercise has a profound impact on our overall wellness. Thus, we must convince ourselves that engaging in any physical activity improves our fitness and must become a priority in our daily routine. The sooner we develop good fitness habits; the sooner we will experience improvements in the quality of our lives.

To understand why exercise is a valuable activity, it is important to learn what happens in our bodies while we exercise. Body movements use the glucose stored in our system to produce energy, which usually comes from proteins and carbohydrates. After depleting glucose, our body requires extra oxygen to create more fuel. Thus, our heart rate increases, and we start to breathe faster and deeper. Adrenaline levels rise, causing our heart to beat faster and circulate more oxygen in our blood, delivering oxygen to all working muscles.

Moderate to vigorous physical activity positively impacts our body in various ways. When we increase the frequency of our workouts, our heart becomes more efficient and enhances blood flow. Regular exercise promotes the development of new blood vessels, causing a reduction in blood pressure.

Increased blood circulation improves brain function, making us more alert and focused immediately after an exercise session. Exercise also promotes brain cell growth, which favors learning and memory, preventing mental decline. As an additional bonus, during exercise sessions, the brain releases endorphins, serotonin, and dopamine, giving us a significant mood boost and making us feel happier and energized.

Health professionals and active people believe that exercise is a natural wonder drug with physical, mental, and emotional benefits. They also know that the results of an active way of life are often accumulated in what might be described as a health bank account, which pays enormous, short, and long-term dividends.

Just as important as saving for a safe and sound retirement, developing the habit of preserving our health will allow us to maintain our independence well into our golden years. Exercise can even turn our biological clock back about a decade.

A person at the peak of health must be active and well-toned, regardless of age. An active person can work, walk, run, jump, swim, dance, lift weights, practice sports, and so on. Movement is the most visible expression of energy. Even people with physical challenges can benefit from movement and exercise.

Types of exercise activities and fitness levels

In general, there are three main types of physical exercise: aerobic, muscle-strengthening, and bone-strengthening, plus two additional categories that include balance and flexibility. Understanding their differences and how they impact your body will help you determine the most appropriate workout that you need to become stronger and fitter.

All forms of exercise have three components: intensity, frequency, and duration. As a rule, it is helpful to mix and alternate low with moderate and high-intensity exercise to maximize health benefits. Our fitness level has an impact on our physical health, and it is directly related to our being sedentary, somewhat active, active, or highly active.

- Aerobic and cardio exercise

Aerobic exercise increases lung efficiency and improves oxygen intake, while cardio exercises make the heart beat faster to pump blood to muscles as they work rhythmically over a continuous period of time. Experts say aerobic and cardio activities are the best way to develop endurance and attain fit and healthy bodies. They include:

· Fast-paced walking	· Jogging
· Swimming	· Rowing
· Biking	· Spinning
· Hiking	· Rollerblading
· Aerobic classes	· Weight training
· Elliptical training	· Playing tennis

Aerobic and cardio activities offer significant health benefits, which are summarized in the following chart:

- Increased lean muscle
- Elevated metabolism
- Increased energy, stamina, and endorphins
- Weight control
- Improved physical appearance
- Decreased intramuscular and subcutaneous fat
- Improved circulation and mental alertness
- Reduced depression, anxiety, and stress
- Increased HDL and lower LDL levels
- More restful sleep

- Muscle-strengthening exercise

This form of exercise trains major muscle groups like shoulders and arms, hips and legs, chest, back and abdomen. It forces muscles to contract against an external force provided by weights, weighted bars, dumbbells, body weight, gravity, bands, etc. These activities include:

- Push-ups and pull-ups
- Curls
- Weightlifting
- Squats
- Shoulder and bench presses
- Spinning

Strength or resistance training helps build, maintain, and preserve muscle and bone mass. These exercises benefit anyone at any age but are especially recommended for people older than 40. They should be an important part of our fitness program to help prevent the loss of lean muscle related to aging.

Strength training makes aerobic activities more efficient by improving our body mechanics in posture, coordination, balance, and joint health. In addition, it reduces the risk of falling in seniors.

Unlike aerobic exercise that can be done daily, strength training should only be done twice or three times a week, for about 30 to 40 minutes, resting about 48 hours between workout sessions to give muscles the opportunity to recover and benefit from the resistance efforts.

Note: it is recommended to warm up before strength training to prevent injuries.

- Bone-strengthening exercise

This is an activity that stimulates bone formation by making us work against gravity. The force generated is produced when our body is in contact with the ground. Bone-strengthening exercises also lower the rate of calcium loss as we get older, reducing the risk of osteoporosis and fractures. Bone-strengthening activities include:

- Stretching
- Brisk Walking
- Hiking
- Dancing
- Jumping Jacks
- Climbing Stairs
- Running
- Playing Golf or Tennis

- Balance and flexibility exercises

These routines help us control a variety of body movements. They improve performance related to coordination, stability, reflexes, speed, and mobility. They also contribute to the prevention of injuries and falls while we are stationary or moving. Balance and flexibility exercises include the following:

- Stretching
- Brisk walking
- Pilates
- Tai chi
- Biking
- Walking backwards
- Standing on one leg
- Yoga
- Dancing
- Playing golf

Although each activity matters when it comes to developing a healthier lifestyle, aerobic and muscle-strengthening exercises offer increased benefits resulting from intensity, frequency, and duration.

Aerobic intensity involves the amount of physical exertion while performing an exercise. For example, a brisk walk requires less physical effort than running. Thus, standing is a low-intensity activity; walking is moderate, and running or jogging are vigorous forms of exercise.

On the other hand, the intensity of muscle-strengthening exercises depends on how much weight a person can lift. Frequency refers to how often an activity is done, and duration depends on how long an activity lasts, including the number of repetitions completed.

A person's fitness level depends on the frequency, intensity, and duration of the activities one does at every stage in life. As we age, our ability to perform vigorous exercise decreases, yet if we want our bodies to continue functioning properly, we must be committed to staying as physically active as possible.

Identifying our fitness level

There are four main adult fitness levels: sedentary, somewhat active, active, and highly active. This classification is based primarily on aerobic activity.

A Sedentary describes someone whose lifestyle involves a lot of sitting and very little physical activity. Being sedentary has serious detrimental health consequences, including obesity, chronic diseases, loss of muscle strength, mental decline, and premature death. Each year, more than 5 million people worldwide die because of ailments associated with physical inactivity. If you are sedentary, you can reduce your health risks by gradually incorporating moderate activity, like walking, into your daily routine.

A somewhat active person engages in some form of moderate or vigorous daily activity but does not meet the basic physical activity guidelines of 150 minutes of moderate or 75 minutes of vigorous exercise per week, as set by the Centers for Disease Control and Prevention. In order to achieve lasting health benefits, you should incorporate exercise into your daily regimen. The average person should aim to walk between 6,000 and 8,000 steps a day.

An active adult usually performs at least 30 minutes of moderate or vigorous activities per day. That is about 100 steps a minute. This person usually meets the target of 150 minutes of moderate or 75 minutes of vigorous exercise per week. Only moderate and vigorous exercise meet our physical activity needs because a regular exercise program is vital for healthy living.

A highly active person does more than 300 minutes of vigorous activity per week and is often considered athletic or highly fit. These individuals learn to enjoy the physical activities they choose and make them a priority in their daily lives. They are disciplined and obtain the maximum health benefits from exercise.

Physical Activity Guidelines for Various Age Groups

As it has been emphasized repeatedly in this wellness manual, exercise provides the foundation for a healthy life for anyone. It is evident that the more active a person is, the better they feel. However, exercise practices vary according to age.

- Children: Parents must encourage children to engage in various forms of physical activity early in their lives. Moms and dads should become active role models themselves to better motivate their children to participate in sports, games, and fun outdoor activities.

A healthy child should do a minimum of 60 minutes of vigorous active play a day. The most common activities recommended for children are hopping, skipping, jumping, running, biking, hiking, tug-of-war games, martial arts, and various sports, depending on the child's preference and physical ability.

Regular exercise will help children build healthy bones and muscles, increase strength and endurance, improve motor skills and coordination, experience emotional and mental well-being, and prevent obesity. One out of three children are overweight or obese, and unless they become sufficiently active, they run the risk of having weight problems their entire lives.

- **Adolescents and young adults**: At this age, people usually are at the peak of physical health. Therefore, this is the ideal time to develop healthy fitness habits for life. Regular exercise routines must become an essential part of their lifestyle. The bodies of adolescents and young adults benefit greatly from a wide variety of aerobic and strength training exercises required to build lean muscle and increase bone density.

Young people usually have a lot of energy which can be used in vigorous activities like running, rowing, boot camp, spinning classes, hiking, practicing sports, or doing high-intensity interval training (HIIT.) They should also walk as often as possible and aim to do about 10,000 steps a day.

Naturally, a high level of stamina usually declines with age, which makes it even more imperative for younger persons to reap the most benefits from exercising and being active early in their lives.

Ideally, adolescents and young adults should exercise frequently, or at least about 300 minutes a week. Regardless of fitness level, they should increase physical activity and reduce the amount of time spent sitting to burn more calories and avoiding weight gain. According to experts, they must stand as often as possible "because sitting can kill them."

Busy schedules should not prevent youth from exercising. Nurturing their body and taking care of their health is just as important as school, job, or other responsibilities. They do not need to go to the gym every day because any activity or sport that gets their heart and lungs pumping fast counts toward their weekly goal. They must find creative ways to include bursts of physical activity into their routine. To get the most benefits out of exercise, everyone has to make physical activity a priority. No excuses!

- **Older adults and seniors**: Although older adults tend to slow down and become more sedentary with age, physical activity is vital for healthy aging. Older people do not have to be frail, sedentary, or overweight because the health benefits of exercise are visible even in people with physical impairments or chronic diseases.

Fitness habits offer almost anyone the possibility of preventing or reducing physical and mental deterioration. Therefore, exercise can lead to better life quality. Staying active into a person's golden years makes a significant contribution to feeling and looking younger and experiencing optimal well-being.

It has been said that exercise adds years to a person's life. Therefore, older adults and seniors should try different kinds of activities to keep moving, such as brisk walking, climbing stairs, yoga, Tai -chi, biking, swimming, dancing, weightlifting, and gardening. These are safe alternatives to increase activity in a daily routine. More fit seniors can choose hiking, jogging, rowing, playing pickleball, tennis, golf, ping-pong, or water volleyball.

Older adults and seniors should do at least 150 minutes of moderate or 75 minutes of vigorous aerobic exercise per week to boost energy levels and maintain a healthy weight. They should also do strength training twice a week to maintain muscle and bone mass. Swimming aerobics can also be a great way to develop strength. Plus, incorporating balance and flexibility exercises will help people in these age groups enhance their mobility and remain independent longer.

Strategies to increase physical activity

Although many people acknowledge the benefits of exercise, some may lack the motivation or the interest to engage in regular physical activity. Others may think that working out demands a great deal of effort and time. Additional factors lead people to have negative attitudes about exercise. They include being overweight, feeling powerless, having a low body image, or any previous unpleasant experiences.

Regardless of the reasons for the lack of exercise, it is evident that developing the habit of being physically active is more difficult for some people than for others. This explains why it is often ignored or eliminated from our daily schedules, even though this practice is empowering and makes us gain control of our well-being.

If done with discipline and dedication, exercise can become a very enjoyable, rewarding, and satisfying activity for everyone. Regular physical activity provides opportunities to have fun, unwind, relax, and be outdoors. These are powerful reasons to make it a priority in our daily lives.

The following recommendations will help increase your motivation to engage in frequent physical activity.

1. Turn your negative attitudes about exercise into a positive mindset. Being physically active will not come naturally to you unless you modify your conscious or unconscious outlook on exercise. To overcome your mental barriers, identify the reasons why you are sedentary.

If you think that exercise is boring, exhausting, or time-consuming, talk to people who are passionate about being fit. They are likely to give you encouragement to become more active. A person's love for exercise is usually highly contagious.

Also, look at images of active people, not to compare yourself with them, but to be inspired by them. Keep in mind that exercise is not another dreadful task on your to-do list but an opportunity to enhance your well-being.

2. Take small steps to challenge yourself to move around more often. If you dislike gyms, cardio equipment, or fitness classes, find ways to increase activity here and there. For example, rather than taking an elevator, use the stairs as often as possible; park your car a bit further or avoid using it when running errands; go for a 10-minute walk in your neighborhood or in a park twice a week. Any time you get up and move, you are making a contribution to your own good health.

You do not need to have a structured exercise program to work out, but you can occasionally try using an exercise machine at home. Start with ten-minute sessions and gradually increase the length of time.

Get a couple of light weights to do arm exercises while you watch TV or as you walk. These simple actions will likely help you gain confidence in your ability to move more frequently. Remember that the human body needs to be in motion and that any physical activity is better than none.

3. Learn to overcome the discomfort of working out in public. It is true that many people feel somewhat intimidated the first time they walk into a gym or a fitness class. They may either be out of shape, afraid of using the equipment properly, unsure about wearing the right clothes, or simply distressed at being surrounded by strangers.

Although being afraid to work out in public is normal, convince yourself that these fears are usually unfounded because most people are focused on their own routines or thoughts as they work out. Furthermore, you will soon realize that many individuals like to welcome and assist newcomers.

4. Find physical activities that you enjoy doing. You are likely to increase your motivation to exercise if you choose routines that fit your interests, abilities, and lifestyle. Avoid getting involved in forms of exercise you find monotonous simply because they seem appropriate or have been recommended to you. Pretending to adjust to an "ideal" plan may end up being another reason to fail.

Once you get tired of an activity in your exercise routine, no amount of determination will help you maintain a long-term commitment to it. Unless that activity is fun and satisfying, try something new. Explore various alternatives until you find the ones that are most worthy of your efforts.

5. Seek adequate support to enhance your exercise motivation and progress. Working with a life coach, a trainer, an exercise partner, or a fitness app is an effective way to jump-start an exercise regimen and to make physical activity a priority. Coaches or trainers will guide, inspire, and make you accountable for your life improvements.

Pairing and committing to exercise with a buddy or a fitness group will encourage you to stay on track and prevent you from skipping an activity. Fitness apps often add variety to a physical routine. They also help you develop a plan that you can follow, create a record of your workouts, and keep track of your progress.

6. Be patient and maintain realistic expectations. Transforming an out-of-shape body is a slow process that takes time and continuous effort. Expecting immediate results from your first attempts will lead to disappointment and discouragement.

Instead of focusing on the visual outcomes of exercise, enjoy the quick psychological effects of an increase in willpower, energy, and well-being. Give yourself credit for the consistency of your fitness efforts. Use these gratifying results to incorporate other healthy behaviors into your life, and the physical rewards will follow. Remember, a few days or weeks may make little difference initially, but many will certainly do!

To keep in mind

- Prolonged sitting and a sedentary lifestyle increase the risk of premature death.

- Physical activity improves our fitness and must become a priority in our daily routine.

- Regular exercise can turn our biological clock back about a decade.

- If done with dedication, exercise can become a very enjoyable, rewarding and satisfying activity.

Questions to reflect on:

1. Do you have an active or a sedentary lifestyle? Explain

2. Do you meet the general exercise requirements for your age group?

3. List three benefits of aerobic or cardio exercises?

4. How often should a person do strength training a week?

5. Does your current fitness level promote good health?

Chapter 6:

Factors that Affect Our Emotional and Mental Health

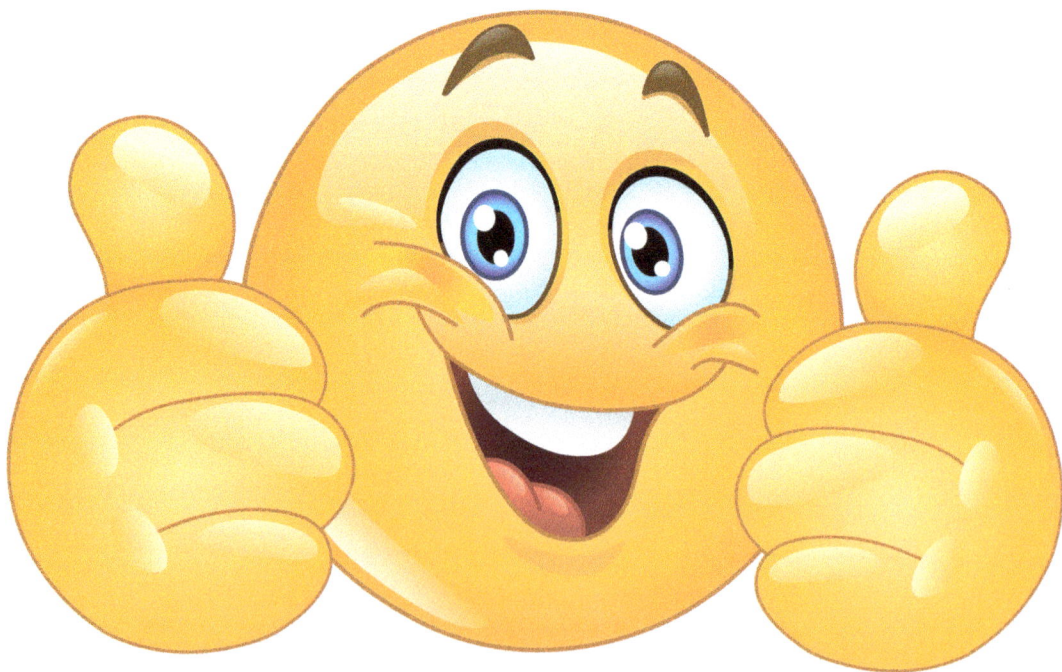

Emotional and mental wellness involves not only being aware of our thoughts, emotions, and behaviors but also managing them effectively. Having emotional and mental wisdom can help us develop a positive outlook, feel good about ourselves, develop nurturing relationships with family, friends, and neighbors, overcome life's ups and downs, and surmount major setbacks when they occur.

The World Health Organization defines mental and emotional wellness as a state of well-being that allows people to realize their abilities, work productively, cope with the normal stresses of life, and contribute to their societies.

Good mental health is vital to psychological, emotional, and social well-being. It is often associated with forward-looking thoughts, satisfying feelings, and meaningful actions. It also means fully engaging with the world and demonstrating enthusiasm for life. Mentally balanced people tend to be physically healthier; good mental health promotes longevity.

In contrast, poor mental health resulting from unhealthy routines, self-destructive attitudes, and inability to overcome hardships damages our well-being. In general, negative thoughts and emotions are toxic. They generate mental noise and are associated with stress, anxiety, sadness, and aggression. Mentally unbalanced people can become depressed and develop eating disorders and addictions, which can cause higher mortality rates.

Being mindful of our emotional health can help us maintain adequate mental hygiene and prevent mental deterioration. However, when mental illness is part of our genetic history, when we cannot lead satisfying and productive lives, or when we fail to savor life's joys, we should seek professional help. Depending on the gravity of our pathologies, we may need the support of a psychiatrist, a psychologist, a counselor, or a health coach.

Visible signs of mental distress that require professional attention:

- Difficulty focusing on daily activities.

- Experiencing extreme emotions like anger, fear, stress, anxiety, or depression.

- Having an ongoing sense of failure, frustration, or hopelessness.

- Experiencing persistent sadness and inability to "shake off the blues."

- Loss or increase of appetite and sleep.

- Feeling extremely pessimistic about the future.

- Being unable to keep going.

While being emotionally and mentally stable does not mean feeling permanently happy or satisfied, emotionally balanced individuals have some common traits that help them gain a sense of control of their lives. They often:

- Take responsibility for what happens to them and for their own actions.
- Learn from previous mistakes and are not victims of their circumstances.
- Are flexible and adapt to new situations by learning to cope with challenges.
- Have strong social connections.
- Acknowledge that life is overall good, rewarding, and meaningful.
- Identify their life purpose and work on their goals with determination.

Every person's life is affected by various types of stressors, conflicts, struggles, and even losses. Our emotional well-being depends mainly on our capacity to respond to those challenges, regardless of what happens to us. Indeed, no one is at the mercy of their circumstances; thus, most of us have the power to construct our own destinies and attain greater well-being.

It has been said that problems build character, making us stronger and more resilient. In contrast, being unable to deal with difficult emotions can lead us to feel moody, angry, resentful, or depressed. Unhealthy responses to difficult emotions can damage the quality of our life and our relationships. By keeping us in survival mode, they can also prevent us from experiencing peace of mind.

Therapists advise us not to ignore or suppress negative thoughts and feelings. Instead, we should transform them by asking ourselves why we feel like we do. It is vital to understand the deeper meaning behind every negative emotion. Unless we acknowledge the causes of our feelings, we cannot change them into positive emotions or actions.

Fortunately, human beings have the enormous capacity to overcome and grow through challenges and find satisfaction and happiness. We can adopt mechanisms that tame our thoughts and restrain our hurtful feelings. The more successful we are in overcoming emotional difficulties, the more motivated we will be to advance on our healthy journeys.

The first step in creating a more fulfilling life is being fully conscious of the kind of existence we really want. This should lead us to determine not only the true sources of personal satisfaction and well-being but also the barriers that hold us back. Although we are sometimes constrained by external forces, in the end, we are ultimately responsible for our decisions and the quality of our life. Most people have the capacity to lead balanced and fulfilling lives.

If we want to thrive, it is essential to take responsibility for our successes and failures, for our happiness and frustrations, for our motivation and discouragement, for our determination to act, and for our self-defeating behaviors. Furthermore, we have a significant impact on the condition of our health, our physical fitness, our attitudes, our relationships, and our life satisfaction.

If any aspect of our existence is not going in the direction of our desires, dreams, and goals, we need to ask ourselves what can be changed or done differently to get better results. In addition, to be successful at any task or undertaking, we must recognize when we are making excuses or finding justifications for any lack of progress.

According to experts, most human beings can learn new behaviors, change their mindsets, adopt healthy habits, overcome addictions, and transform their lives. In other words, we are capable of increasing our mental and emotional intelligence by accepting that just about anything can be accomplished with the right amount of determination and motivation.

Factors That Interfere with Our Mental Balance

1. Having low self-esteem

Self-esteem is our self-image and corresponds to the value we place on ourselves. It often has a direct impact on the choices we make. A high sense of self-worth makes us do meaningful things, which in turn reinforces our self-image; low self-esteem leads us to be stuck in the cycle of devaluing ourselves and feeling inferior to others, which in turn, damages our image even further. Higher levels of happiness are associated with good self-esteem.

Being dissatisfied with ourselves has serious consequences. It can provoke poor academic and job performance, alcohol and drug use, and disordered eating, or it can even bring about criminal behavior.

The most common causes of low self-esteem are:

- Negligent parents who do not provide children with adequate care, attention, and a loving family.
- Trauma, bullying, or abuse, whether emotional, physical, or sexual.
- Poor body image, which makes us feel unattractive and self-conscious.
- Unrealistic goals that foster negative emotions of failure and powerlessness.
- Past or present bad choices and risky behaviors, which make us feel shame and dislike ourselves.

Given that self-esteem is a state of mind, you can improve yours by identifying the sources of your dissatisfaction and changing the behaviors that make you feel uncomfortable. Commit to giving yourself the care and attention you deserve and learn to manage difficult emotions. Getting the support of family and friends, along with professional counseling, is highly recommended.

2. Having stress and anxiety

Stress and anxiety are perhaps the most pervasive and common mental issues in our fast-paced world. Stress is a negative response caused by the desire to complete something yet being unable to get it done. Anxiety is the sense of uneasiness, distress, or dread experienced before a significant event in our life.

When we feel stressed or anxious, our brain senses danger and triggers the fight or flight response mechanism. This generates an automatic reaction in our nervous system to prepare our body to do battle or run away. As a result, our body releases hormones and chemicals designed to help us respond to the threat. Adrenaline and cortisol are two examples.

An increase in adrenaline and cortisol, which is called the stress hormone, raises our breathing, blood pressure, and heart rate. Both hormones give us a burst of energy to respond appropriately to a dangerous situation. However, this survival mechanism can also make us less rational and more reactive and aggressive.

While stress and anxiety are natural conditions in life, an excessive and prolonged state of stress and anxiety is highly detrimental to our physical and mental health. Research shows that cortisol prevents the brain from making new neurons and nerve cells, causing premature aging of the brain.

Cortisol can also elevate blood pressure and increase the risk of a heart attack or stroke. Long-term exposure to cortisol can have a negative effect on the immune system, leaving us more vulnerable to viral infections and various illnesses. It also contributes to weight gain, high cholesterol, diabetes, and even hair loss.

It needs to be stated that not all stress is negative or harmful and that some moderate levels could even enhance our productivity and creativity. Also, the way we view stress and handle stressors is key for it to become a minor or major cause of concern.

Stress can be acute, post-traumatic, or chronic. Acute stress is experienced for a short period of time, and our body recovers rapidly from it. Post-Traumatic Stress Disorder (PTSD) often lasts a few months or longer. It is a condition of persistent mental and emotional stress resulting from a severe psychological shock, injury, or traumatic experience. Its symptoms include recurring flashbacks, severe anxiety, uncontrollable thoughts, and nightmares about the event. Most people recover from it with time, self-care, or effective treatment.

Chronic stress is experienced over a long period of time due to internal or external factors such as work overload, poverty, financial troubles, toxic relationships, etc. This constant stress is very detrimental to our health and can lead to physical and mental exhaustion and illness.

The key to controlling chronic stress and anxiety is identifying the factors or situations that cause it, whether at home, work, relationships, or finances. And even though we may not be able to alter most of the circumstances of our daily lives, we should try to keep stressors under control. On the other hand, a therapist can help us identify stressors and develop coping tools.

- Academic, professional, or financial pressures
- Major life changes
- Loss, grief, illness
- Fear and uncertainty
- Unrealistic expectations and perfectionism
- Concerns with body image
- Relationship difficulties and emotional problems
- Challenges balancing personal, social, and professional lives

The most common symptoms of stress are:

- Difficulty concentrating and thinking clearly
- Increased irritability, frustration, angry outbursts
- Feeling overwhelmed and out of control
- Obsessive thinking, nervousness, depression, and sadness
- Chest pain, racing heart, and rapid breathing
- Upset stomach, constipation, or diarrhea
- Changes in sleep and/or eating patterns
- Fatigue and lack of energy and motivation
- Substance use to cope, including tobacco, alcohol, and illegal drugs

Note: To learn more about active ways to cope with stress, refer to the section Relaxation: Relieving Stress Naturally and Effectively, in this book.

3. Experiencing breakups, losses, and traumas

In the life of most people, there are events such as the death of a loved one, an accident, a natural disaster, a terrorist attack, a pandemic, domestic violence, a divorce, or a job loss that often have a lasting impact on our mental health. As a result, we may experience distressing reactions that prevent us from engaging in our daily activities or from maintaining a positive state of mind.

Acknowledging that some hardships may be extremely painful, we must find ways to cope with grief and adjust to unexpected changes. Challenging events in life can become profound learning opportunities, and they can even trigger positive changes. However, when the impact of these adversities is too severe, seeking professional help is compelling.

Some strategies that can facilitate our recovery from a severe crisis include problem-solving coping and emotional coping. Problem-solving coping focuses on finding ways to act on a situation, while emotional coping is centered on managing our responses or reactions to alleviate the hurt. Problem-solving coping includes the following steps:

- Analyzing and evaluating the situation
- Thinking of ways to handle the conflict in a constructive manner
- Getting advice from someone who has had a similar experience
- Planning a set of actions to be followed
- Putting forth the best efforts to tackle the problem

Emotional coping may require finding support from loved ones or guidance from experts and making a conscious decision to move forward. The main objective of emotional coping is to distract the mind with relaxing or pleasant activities to release tension.

Activities that can facilitate emotional recovery include:

- Sharing our feelings with others
- Developing an understanding and acceptance of the event
- Finding a silver lining in the situation
- Engaging in various types of physical exercise
- Practicing relaxation activities like meditation, yoga, or massage therapy
- Getting outside and spending time in nature

4. Having chronic illness, debilitating pain, or a disability

Major health issues, long-term or life-threatening illnesses, and disabilities can have detrimental effects on our mental well-being. They often impair functioning and cause frustration, anxiety, despair, and unhappiness. Furthermore, the prevalence of chronic ailments can lead to severe mental damage and depression.

It is well-known that there is a reciprocal relationship between our physical and mental wellness. Indeed, it has been stated that a healthy body supports a healthy mind. Evidently, it is difficult to maintain a balanced life when our body lets us down. Poor physical health prevents us from having the motivation and the energy to engage in regular daily activities, maintain personal autonomy, have mobility, and keep a positive outlook.

Given that many chronic conditions are preventable, we should monitor our health to identify health risk factors as early as possible. Their minor or major effects should be mitigated through adequate treatment and medication, pain therapies, and targeted lifestyle changes. By reducing the burden of these conditions, we can regain good health and boost our mental well-being.

Ideally, we can all improve our health and increase our life expectancy. Furthermore, most of us have the potential to develop and maintain thriving bodies to serve us well into our golden years. This is certainly the best alternative to enjoy productive lives and avoid chronic pain, mental suffering, high medical expenses, medication side effects, etc.

It is worth repeating over and over that the secret to optimal physical and mental health is very simple: healthy eating, regular physical activity, resting, managing stress levels, and developing strong social connections. When taking care of our bodies becomes a priority, we are making the best investment in our own well-being and happiness.

5. Having unwanted habits, compulsive behaviors, and addictions

Our habits and behaviors are signs of our mental health. In general, most people are born habit or addiction-free and in good mental health. Therefore, most habits and addictions are artificially created by our thoughts and reinforced by our actions. They often hide discomfort, inner conflicts, and dissatisfaction. Unfortunately, various life experiences can lead us to develop bad habits, compulsions, or addictions.

It is important to understand that a habit is a repetitive action that generates an automatic response in the brain. Everyone has good habits that serve us well, like being early risers, along with undesirable behaviors that we wish we did not have, like nail biting or having a phone dependency. The brain makes no distinction between positive and negative habits, and once a routine becomes automatic, it is difficult to override.

Bad habits usually make us feel unhappy or uncomfortable. They can have a negative impact on the quality of our life, and they can become obstacles to what we really want for ourselves. Evidently, some habits are more difficult to break than others, but we should not hesitate to modify poor habits that affect our health or frustrate us.

A compulsion is an uncontrollable or obsessive urge to do something resulting from fear or anxiety. People with Obsessive-Compulsive Disorder (OCD) may feel compelled to perform some rituals repeatedly, or they may experience intrusive thoughts that can be very distressing. Common compulsions include constant handwashing and counting, being obsessed with cleanliness, and having a need for symmetry.

Addictions are destructive behaviors characterized by an out-of-control need to do something. Addicts depend on a substance or behavior to experience pleasure or find relief from discomfort. The pleasure or relief experienced is so strong that they disregard the negative consequences of their actions, which often include family and social rejection, job loss, financial ruin, legal troubles, homelessness, physical discomfort, and others.

Because many addictions lead to disability and death, they are considered diseases in the medical world. They often have a devastating impact on people's health, careers, relationships, and lives.

Although not all bad habits become addictions, there is a fine line separating them. Some habits can become addictive behaviors. For instance, social drinking can gradually turn into alcoholism, or poor eating habits can lead to binge or compulsive eating. Once a harmful behavior becomes compulsive, it is imperative to seek counseling and adequate medical treatment.

Fortunately, most people have the capacity to overcome poor habits, compulsions, and addictions. Indeed, and as it has been stated before, most of us are capable of successful behavioral changes. To start, addictions and compulsions are treatable conditions, though they require professional assistance in the form of therapy and medication.

Changing undesirable habits, on the other hand, may or may not require counseling, depending on the person. The task of breaking habits can be implemented with enough motivation, support, and good reversal training strategies. Making the decision to modify a harmful behavior for good can lead to achieving a more meaningful and satisfying life.

Note: To learn more about breaking bad habits, refer to the section Changing Undesirable Habits for Better Health, in this book.

6. Fostering hatred, anger, and resentment

Hatred, anger, and resentment are some of the most common human emotions, but when they take control of our minds, they generate more negative feelings. Grudges and bitterness are destructive because they force us to carry insidious and heavy psychological baggage within us. The seeds of these emotions poison our lives and have detrimental effects on our health.

We tend to experience anger and hostility when we feel wronged, hurt, or attacked by another person. These are natural responses to any kind of physical, emotional, or sexual aggression. They usually lead us to either seek retaliation or distance ourselves from the aggressor. However, allowing animosity and hostility to overpower us will force us to be consumed by them.

Anger, hatred, and resentment impair our capacity to reason and make proper decisions. They cause great suffering and compel us to harm others. They also keep us trapped in a cycle of pain, unable to experience peace.

Positive anger can be a constructive force when it is motivated by empathy and compassion. It is an impulse that promotes change. Healthy levels of anger are acceptable, especially when we realize that we are not being treated fairly, respectfully, or with consideration. Yet, constantly feeling upset breeds negative consequences.

Various clinical studies have documented the damaging physical and mental effects of being obsessed over an offense or aggression. Being locked in anger and frustration puts our cardiovascular system at risk of heart disease and high blood pressure, impairs our immune system, provokes ulcers and other ailments, and increases depression.

Given that these emotions come from within us, we have the choice of ruminating on the hurtful event, or liberating ourselves from the misery and the transgressor, by learning to forgive. Forgiveness is the only way to overcome our feelings of victimhood. It allows us to positively channel our anger and restore our inner peace, serenity, and happiness.

If you are unable to tame your anger, hatred, or resentment, you must seek counseling or find a way to move forward. Here are some ideas to help you manage your anger:

- Be mindful of and accept your hurt feelings
- Ask yourself why you are having hateful thoughts
- Do something relaxing to calm yourself down
- When you are calm, think of ways to effectively deal with the issue
- If the problem is beyond your control, change your mindset about it
- Share your feelings with someone who can give you objective advice
- Think of the impact these emotions have on your mental health
- Train your mind to focus on the positive aspects of your life
- If possible, choose to walk the path of forgiveness

Forgiveness has different meanings and implications for people. It does not mean denying or repressing your anger and bitterness. It does not entail condoning abusive behavior or accepting victimhood. It does not even include reconciliation with the person that has hurt us, though this is an optional step in the forgiving process.

Reconciliation begins with accepting that suffering is ingrained in the human condition and that no one is immune to pain. Perhaps you can adopt a somewhat benevolent perspective and be willing to let go of your animosity if you assess the situation from the offender's point of view. It must be recognized that the nature of certain aggressions may still be unforgivable.

Steps in the forgiveness process:

- Consider the benefits of forgiveness to facilitate your healing
- Remember the times you hurt someone and were forgiven
- Learn about how other people have successfully forgiven others
- Determine the symptoms of your emotional distress
- Put your emotions in writing, describing the harm caused to you
- Look for a therapist or join a support group
- Make a conscious decision to move from pain to forgiveness

Forgiveness can bring about several psychological and physical benefits, such as:

- Greater mental well-being and restored positive thinking
- Reduced anxiety, hostility, and stress
- Improved capacity to manage conflict
- Healed relationships
- Lower blood pressure and enhanced heart health
- Stronger immune system

7. Experiencing insomnia and other sleep disorders

Insomnia, disturbed sleep and sleep deprivation are very frequent among the general population, but these sleep disturbances may contribute to the development of some mental disorders like depression and anxiety.

Practicing healthy sleep habits increases our ability to get restorative, restful, and uninterrupted sleep. Therefore, we must become aware of the impact that our daily routines have on the quality of our sleep. There is no doubt that sleep plays a vital role in our mental and emotional well-being.

Insomnia is a sleep disorder that prevents people from falling asleep smoothly and staying asleep throughout the night. A person suffering from insomnia often takes more than 30 minutes to fall asleep and may not manage to reach a stage of deep sleep. Deep sleep is essential for physical and mental recovery and development. It helps us process information and make better decisions. It also contributes to memory consolidation and learning.

Insomnia can be acute when it lasts a few days or a few weeks. This temporary disturbance is usually caused by stress or physical discomfort. In contrast, chronic stress can last more than three months (and might be experienced more than three days a week.) It may result from poor sleep habits, substance abuse, medication, anxiety, medical problems, or any mental disorder.

Acute or chronic insomnia has serious negative consequences for us. A lack of sleep prevents us from functioning adequately and reduces our productivity. Restless sleep makes us feel drowsy, irritable, and moody. It causes difficulty concentrating on tasks, daytime sleepiness, and exhaustion. Maintaining adequate sleep hygiene can greatly reduce the risk of experiencing insomnia, improving our overall health.

One of the most effective ways to treat insomnia is called Cognitive Behavioral Therapy (CBT.) It is a type of psychotherapy that focuses on altering thoughts and behaviors that prevent sleep, learning techniques for stress reduction and relaxation, and facilitating sleep schedule management.

Here is a list of healthy tips given by experts that will promote restful sleep and prevent chronic insomnia:

- Keep a consistent sleep schedule throughout the entire week and on vacation.
- Get between 7 to 8 hours of sleep per night.
- Get enough sunlight exposure in the morning.
- Exercise regularly and follow a healthy diet.
- Establish a relaxing bedtime routine (doing guided meditation, taking a warm bath, practicing slow breathing, doing puzzles, or listening to soothing music.)
- Make your bedroom comfortable, relaxing, and quiet.
- Reduce exposure to bright light and noise in the evening.
- Avoid using blue-light electronic devices at least an hour before bed.
- Have a light, early dinner.
- Do not consume caffeine late in the afternoon or in the evening.
- Reduce alcohol and fluid intake before bedtime.
- Go to bed as soon as you start feeling sleepy.
- Get out of bed if you do not fall asleep in 20 minutes.
- Do a short relaxing activity (away from an electronic device) before returning to bed.
- Reduce stress and worry as much as possible.
- Identify your insomnia triggers.
- Join an insomnia support group online.

When analyzing your sleep patterns consider sleep duration and sleep quality. They both matter. You can learn what causes your insomnia by paying attention to your routines. Self-awareness may help you improve your sleep habits.

If you continue to have sleep issues or have a sleep disorder, share your concerns with your doctor or a sleep specialist to determine the right course of action and find an appropriate treatment.

Additional serious sleep disorders you may need to be aware of include sleep apnea, restless leg syndrome, and narcolepsy, among others. Sleep apnea makes the body reduce or stop breathing during sleep due to obstructions in the airways.

Restless leg syndrome causes very uncomfortable sensations in the legs and an uncontrollable urge to move them. These symptoms become more severe in night, making it difficult to fall asleep.

Narcolepsy is a disorder characterized by daytime drowsiness and exhaustion, which provoke involuntary sleepiness. People with narcolepsy can fall asleep anywhere and anytime.

8. Struggling with depression

Depression has become an epidemic mood disorder experienced by about 264 million people, and it is the second-leading cause of death worldwide. This illness causes great emotional suffering manifested in persistent sadness and lack of interest in pleasurable activities. It is a difficult ailment to endure and a potential risk factor for dementia and heart disease.

There is an important difference between sadness and depression. While sadness is a natural and necessary human emotion, depression can severely affect a person's ability to function and achieve a satisfying life. Its disabling symptoms disturb important areas in a person's life, such as thinking, concentration, motivation, sleep, and appetite. In addition, they promote hopelessness, frustration, and grief.

If you feel depressed, consult a mental health specialist or your medical doctor without delay. When left untreated, depression can get worse, resulting in major emotional and behavioral problems. And even though it usually requires long-term treatment, most people with mild or severe depression can recover with the help of antidepressant medication and psychotherapy.

Depression has social, psychological, and biological causes. It can be triggered by stressful life events and unresolved conflicts that lead to prolonged psychological stress. It can also result from a temporary family crisis, a job loss, or even unrealistic expectations.

Low self-esteem, self-neglect, phobias, alcohol or drug abuse, and panic attacks are often associated with depression. Furthermore, depression can be genetic. That is, some people can be born with a predisposition toward the disease, especially if they have relatives who endure the same condition. There are four common types of depression:

Seasonal affective depression. It is a type of mild depression resulting from changes in seasons. The low mood shifts often begin in the fall and increase in the winter months due to a reduction of sunlight. Many people tend to feel down when the days get shorter, resulting in decreased levels of serotonin. An overproduction of melatonin increases sleepiness. Furthermore, deficits in vitamin D also contribute to winter blues.

Persistent depressive disorder or dysthymia. It is a long-lasting, though less severe, kind of depression. It allows people to function daily, but they still feel unable to overcome their gloomy moods and experience joy.

Major depression. It is a permanent state of dissatisfaction, sadness, or unhappiness and lack of interest in pleasurable activities. It is usually followed by eating and sleeping disturbances. Thoughts of death and suicide may be experienced.

Bipolar or manic-depressive disorder. It involves extreme uncontrolled mood swings in which episodes of severe depression and irritability appear after states of great euphory, enthusiasm, energy, and hyperactivity.

In general, people can have occasional episodes of mild depression that can last a few days. However, experiencing persistent blues for more than two years can turn into a severe disorder. Beware of the following signs of depression:

- Feelings of sadness, unhappiness, and a sense of emptiness or hopelessness
- Lack of interest in doing regular and enjoyable activities
- Lack of energy, exhaustion, and inability to perform even small tasks
- Mental fog and inability to concentrate or think clearly
- Sleeping issues, either with insomnia or oversleeping
- Eating problems due to loss of appetite or overeating
- Extreme irritability, agitation, or frustration
- Thoughts of death or suicide

Treatment for depression often includes medication, therapy, and healthy lifestyle choices. To start, become as informed as possible about your case and treatment options. They often depend on your case and the severity of your symptoms. Be ready to experiment with various options and medications before you find the one that works for you. Be patient because it can take time and determination to find the most effective treatment for you. Finally, do not rely only on medications, and be ready to practice self-care.

Things you can do for yourself to treat and/or prevent depression:

1. **Do regular exercise** to effectively improve your mental health (For maximum results, do 30 to 60 minutes of aerobic activity five times a week.)

2. **Have healthy nutrition** (Avoid processed foods, reduce sugar and salt intake.)

3. **Take Omega-3 fatty acids** (from food and quality supplements; about 2.5 grams daily.)

4. **Sleep well** to improve emotional well-being and reduce depression symptoms.

5. **Increase dietary fiber** to improve microbiome quality and enhance mental health.

6. **Get regular sunlight exposure** (at least 15 minutes of the morning sun.)

7. **Develop strong social connections** with family and friends and reduce isolation.

- Mental and emotional wellness involves being fully engaged with others and feeling enthusiasm for life.

- Excessive stress and anxiety are highly detrimental to physical and mental health.

- Good sleep habits are essential for physical and mental recovery and well-being.

- Depression causes emotional suffering and affects a person's ability to function and enjoy life.

Questions to reflect on:

1. Do you consider yourself a mentally balanced person? Explain

2. From the list provided at the beginning of this chapter, can you identify any signs of distress that you experience regularly?

3. What mechanisms do you use to cope with your daily stressors?

4. Based on the reading, what urgent behaviors should you modify to improve your mental health?

Chapter 7:

Understanding Addictions and Compulsive Behaviors

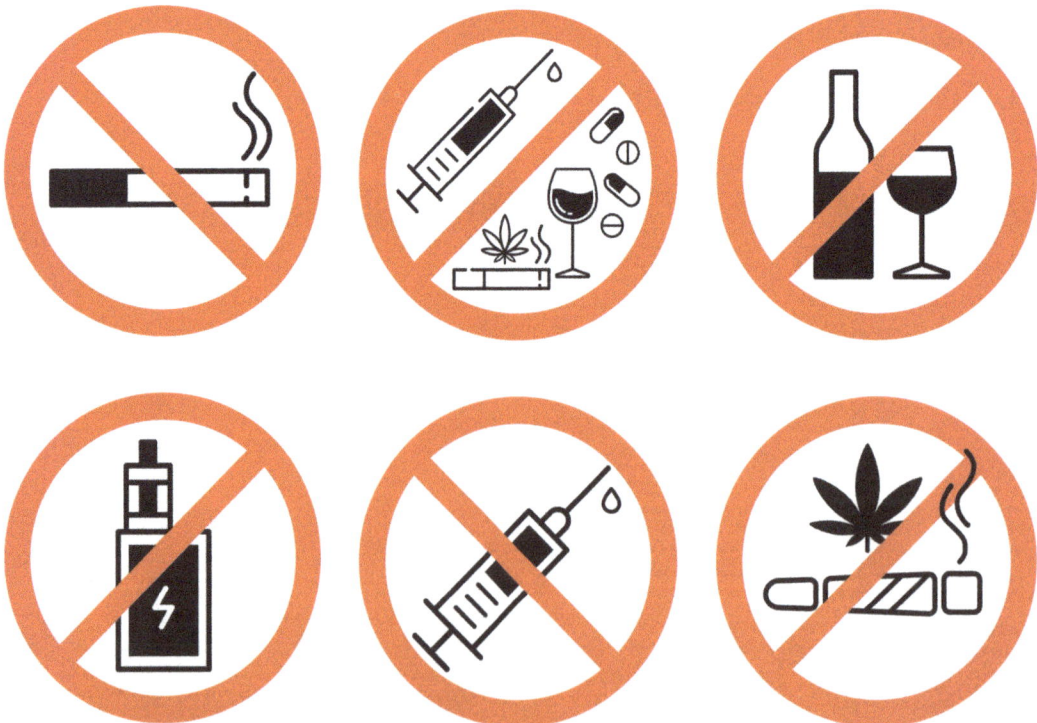

According to the latest United Nations World Report, there are about 270 million people who use drugs globally. Over the past decade, opioid death rates have increased by about 71% worldwide, and almost a million deaths due to opioid overdose have occurred in the United States over the past 20 years. On the other hand, alcohol kills 2.8 million people every year globally, causing cancer, heart problems, homicides, suicides, and road accidents. Drug problems and alcohol abuse are major health concerns everywhere.

Part of the process of fostering wisdom should lead people to a deeper understanding of the power of addictive drugs and addictive behaviors before they fall into their vicious trap. By learning how addictions work, everyone can contribute to preventing this epidemic from seizing their lives and those of their loved ones.

To start, it must be acknowledged that never using drugs or falling into addictive behaviors is better, safer, and wiser than freeing oneself from the grip of addiction. Various substances and behaviors can trap intelligent, educated, good, decent people in a roller coaster of chemical or behavioral dependency, preventing them from leading sane, balanced lives. Moreover, even though many individuals can have successful recoveries, the possibility of relapse is always present. The relapse rate among drug abusers seeking treatment is very high.

Teens are especially vulnerable to falling into addictions, and they, along with young adults, account for the largest group of drug users. Unfortunately, their brains are not fully developed, particularly the front regions that control risky behaviors and impulses. While every area of the brain is responsible for tasks like managing emotions and critical thinking, *as each region matures, it strengthens a person's abilities in the tasks related to that region. Adolescence is a critical time in brain development.*

Substance abuse during adolescence may interrupt the natural course of brain maturation and key processes of brain growth. It has been associated with alterations in brain structure and function. Adolescents who use addictive substances need a great deal of support from caring adults, school counselors, teachers, mentors, therapists, doctors, and peers to stop them from developing full-blown addiction problems.

Addictions are chronic, progressive diseases that can go into remission, but addicts are never completely cured until they break the cycle of use permanently. Drugs and addictive substances and behaviors alter the brain's normal chemical balance and change how the different areas of the brain interact with one another. Over time, the brain adapts and makes the sought-after substance or activity less pleasurable.

A healthy brain usually rewards healthy behaviors like eating well, exercising, and interacting with others, encouraging us to repeat those actions. It is also wired to make us react when we experience fear or danger. Furthermore, the front region of our brain helps us evaluate the results of our actions. However, repeated use of drugs damages the reward and decision-making centers of our brains.

One of the most significant imbalances caused by addictions is related to the release of natural feel-good chemicals like dopamine, serotonin, and endorphins. They contribute to our mental well-being and make us feel energetic, euphoric, happy, and calm naturally. However, as people develop addictions, their brain is flooded with dopamine and other chemicals. Being overwhelmed, the brain responds by producing less dopamine or eliminating dopamine receptors, leading to depression, anxiety, psychosis, and other mental disorders.

An addiction involves an intense craving for something, a loss of control over the decision to use it, a continuous dependency on the substance or behavior, and lifestyle dysfunction resulting from drug use or practice. It also leads to severe emotional distress when the substance is not available. Although every substance or behavior affects the brain in a different way, their abuse often causes similar adverse consequences that include hurting families and losing jobs.

Causes of addiction and risk factors

Several genetic, psychological, and environmental factors increase someone's possibility of developing substance abuse disorders or addictions. For instance:

- A person's genes or a family history of addiction

- Growing up in a dysfunctional environment (experiencing neglect and emotional or sexual abuse

- Peer and school life pressures (struggles with schoolwork, fear of being excluded and/or bullied

- Psychological and mental problems like depression or bipolar disorder

- Low self-esteem

- High-stress lifestyle

Types of Addiction

Addictions can be physical, psychological, or both. They are classified into two main groups: chemical and behavioral. Chemical addictions involve the abuse and dependency on substances, while behavioral addictions, also called impulse control disorders, involve compulsive actions that are carried out repeatedly and interfere with normal living.

Here is a list of the most frequently abused substances and behavioral addictions:

Chemical Addictions	Behavioral Addictions
Alcohol and Tobacco	Over/undereating
Cannabis (marijuana)	Sex and pornography
Prescription medicines and painkillers	Video games
Opioids, heroin	Internet/social media/phone
Cocaine	Gambling
Methamphetamine	Compulsive shopping
Barbiturates and hallucinogens	Workaholism

Denial is a psychological defense mechanism used by most addicts to minimize their problems. It is a form of self-deception that precludes an individual from confronting their reality even when the signs of trouble are obvious to anyone else. Unfortunately, this attitude can become a serious obstacle to seeking help and starting the recovery process before the situation gets out of hand.

The following are warning signs of addiction resulting from substance use or addictive behavior:

- Trouble managing work, school, or personal responsibilities
- Relationship difficulties with family, friends, or coworkers
- A person not seeming like themselves anymore
- Withdrawal or keeping secrets from family and friends
- Loss of interest in activities that the person used to enjoy
- The decline in personal grooming and hygiene
- Mood swings from extreme emotional highs to lows
- Temper flareups, irritability, anxiety, or depression
- Appearing defensive when asked about substance use or behavior
- Severe changes in sleeping habits
- Changes in eating habits, including weight loss or gain
- Muddled thinking and memory problems
- Financial difficulties and/or problems with the law
- Stealing or selling belongings to be able to afford addictive substances
- Use of addictive substances to forget problems or to relax
- Risky substance use, like driving or working while using it

Beware of the following symptoms. If you experience them, seek help immediately:

- Cravings intense enough to affect your ability to think about other things
- A need to use more of the substance to experience the same effects
- Unease or discomfort if you cannot easily access the substance
- Inability to stop using the substance
- Withdrawal symptoms (feeling sick or shaky) when you try to quit

Treatment to end the cycle of addiction

Recovery from dependency issues starts when a person is determined to overcome an addiction. Although some people are successful in quitting addictions on their own, most people need medical support during this gradual, lengthy process to begin the path of recovery.

There is no universal treatment that cures all addictions. Addiction treatment is highly personalized and often requires the support of the individual's community or family. Treatment methods depend on the type of addiction, a person's needs, and the options they can afford.

Since addiction is a chronic condition that has various psychological and physical effects, finding an effective rehabilitation center and /or treatment can take time and can be complicated. Also, each substance or behavior addiction requires different management techniques.

Treatment modalities may include:

Medically supervised detoxification to reduce substance cravings and withdrawal symptoms.

Behavioral counseling to identify substance abuse triggers and modify harmful thoughts, regulate emotions, learn to cope with crises, and improve relationships, among others.

Peer support groups made up of people who encourage addicts to advance in the recovery journey.

Group counseling to establish relationships with sober individuals and improve interpersonal skills.

Family therapy to heal wrecked family relationships and rebuild trust among its members.

Wellness counseling to prevent relapse and promote physical, emotional, mental, and spiritual well-being.

- Substance abuse is associated with severe alterations in brain structure and function.

- Drugs reduce the brain's capacity to release natural feel-good chemicals like dopamine, serotonin, and endorphins.

- Addictions can be physical or chemical and psychological or behavioral.

- Denial is a psychological defense mechanism used by most addicts to minimize their drug problems or compulsion.

- Recovery from dependency issues starts when a person is determined to overcome an addiction.

Questions to reflect on:

1. Why is substance abuse during adolescence more detrimental to a person's health?

2. What is the difference between physical and psychological addictions?

3. If you have an addiction, are you determined to overcome your dependency and seek professional help?

4. What treatment modality would work best for you? Why?

Chapter 8:

Changing Undesirable Habits for Better Health

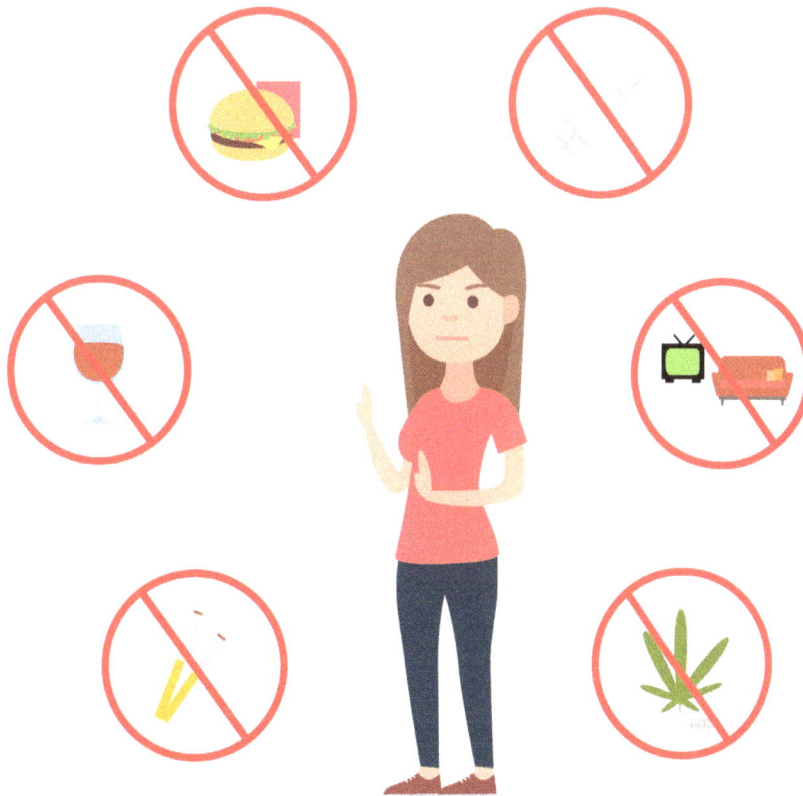

All habits begin with thoughts, which are reinforced every time we give in to cravings and urges. Thus, to achieve behavioral changes, we need to understand the role our mind plays in regulating our routines.

Human beings are endowed with a lower, unintelligent brain responsible for most essential functions to keep us alive. Our lower brain focuses mostly on automatic survival behaviors. In contrast, our higher brain is capable of superior reasoning and sensitivity. It oversees our rational thinking and thoughtful decision-making.

This explains why our mind can get us in trouble, but it can also lead us to perform great endeavors. So, while we may feel powerless or defeated by a bad habit or addiction, our inner wisdom can help us find the right approach to overcome annoying and harmful behaviors.

Knowledge and awareness can empower us in the process of making better life choices. As we gain an understanding of the nature of our habits or addictions, we can become more conscious of their damaging effects. We also come to the realization that settling for bad habits forces us to lead mediocre lives.

Urges are inner thoughts and loud voices that compel us to act in a certain way. They often convey untrue needs, which seek to deprive us of the freedom to make wise decisions. Therefore, we must identify their negative messages to avoid interacting with and being controlled by them.

We can change a poor habit by learning to dismiss its temporary urges. Giving these impulses full attention will make them stronger while managing to ignore them will reduce their frequency. The more someone is exposed to a behavior, the more it is internalized. It has been said that we become what we repeatedly do.

There are various reasons why we let our lower brain control our will and continue being stuck or defeated by our urges. First, we may feel unable to step out of our comfort zone to gain mastery of our minds. Second, we may lack the motivation, discipline, and conviction to change. Third, the behavior we wish to modify is part of a system that keeps our life going for us, even if it harms us.

Often, our lifestyle choices are driven by what gives us more pleasure and relaxation or by what shields us from painful emotions. Thus, an important step in a changing process is to identify the purpose of the unwanted drive in our life. As we understand the factors that lie behind our urge, we will be able to gradually learn to overcome it rather than surrender to its demands. Here is a list of common unwanted habits:

• Overeating	• Snacking on junk food
• Not setting time to exercise	• Not getting enough sleep
• Phone dependency	• Spending too much time online
• Caffeine or stimulant dependency	• Not drinking enough water
• Alcohol overdrinking	• Practicing unprotected sex
• Not using sun protection	• Speeding
• Procrastination	• Being pessimistic

Our inner wisdom can feed us nutritious thoughts to extinguish unhealthy habits and point us toward the right choices for us. It can also give us the power to overcome our weaknesses and to learn from our mistakes.

Overcoming a difficult habit usually takes time, effort, determination, and perseverance. It also entails finding an adequate individual approach, which may or may not rely on seeking professional counseling.

Unfortunately, there is no certified prescription or guaranteed universal method to controlling undesirable behaviors, although a lot of advice is available online or at bookstores. Given that some recommendations work better for certain people than for others, you must identify the most effective course of action for you and your circumstances.

Here are some of the most common suggestions given by experts to actively engage in habit recovery or healing:

1. Identify the attitudes and behaviors that hurt you and others or that hinder your growth. In general, the desire to break a bad habit happens either when you feel emotional discomfort and dissatisfaction or when your behavior causes problems in your relationships with others.

Carry out a personal evaluation of what makes you unhappy and reflect on your need for a behavioral change. Often, self-awareness awakens the call for change. Do not dismiss or run away from these emotions. Also, try not to be defensive when someone who cares about you brings up concerns related to the things that you do. Constructive opinions, advice, and feedback can be beneficial to your health and development.

2. Make a list of some compelling reasons you may have to change the habit. Be as honest as possible when you do this self-evaluation. Think of the main benefits that committing to modifying a behavior will bring you and perhaps your loved ones. Consider the risks regarding your current behavior. Review your notes whenever you are prone to give up on your improvement efforts. They will reinforce your determination to move forward.

3. Learn to develop a positive mindset and self-talk to facilitate change. Stay away from discouraging beliefs or negative attitudes such as "I can't do it," "I always fail," "It is too hard," or "change is impossible for me," among others. Replace any negative thought that curbs your motivation, energy, or enthusiasm. Positive self-talk may include ideas like:

I have the power to change my habit.
This change will enrich my life in various ways.
I am worthy of my efforts to change.
I have faith in my ability to improve myself.
I commit myself to becoming the best version of myself.
I can learn to make the right choices for myself.
This is the right moment to change my harmful behavior.
I want to set a good example for others to follow.
Add your own ideas...

4. Create a simple, doable plan with concrete steps, actions, and/or strategies to follow. Implementing change is never easy, but establishing a clear path that gets you from where you are to where you want to be will facilitate this process. State specific goals in a concise way. For example, rather than having a broad objective like "to get in better shape," you may want to state it as "lose 4 pounds per month by going to the gym 3 times a week and walking for 30 minutes twice a week."

94

The challenge to change your behavior should be as deliberate as possible. It entails controlling factors that favor or interfere with the expected results, monitoring your progress toward your goals, adjusting actions and strategies accordingly, and even modifying the original plan to make it more achievable.

As you undertake a healing journey, rely on your road map to point you in the right direction and develop appropriate attitudes for change. Change does not result from wishful thinking; it only happens when you do the hard work needed for success and when you advance with conscious determination on the path of your goals.

5. Give top priority to your habit-changing efforts over other daily responsibilities. Although many people are prone to sacrifice their personal goals when their agendas get hectic, you ought to give yours the importance they deserve, or you will likely fail to achieve the expected results. Failure happens when you let your job or family obligations push your initiative for improvement back. When life gets in the way of your goals, remember the impact they will have on your overall health and well-being.

Implementing a positive change in your life demands your full commitment and attention. Thus, the steps in your plan of action must be incorporated into your daily routines. Keep in mind that long-term sustained change does not happen quickly and that it may take a minimum of 30 or 40 days for a new habit to be wired into your memory.

Quitting whenever you encounter an obstacle should not be an option. Beware, your lower brain will attempt to sabotage your efforts at every opportunity by giving you multiple excuses and distractions to cling to the status quo. Yet do not expect to change a habit if you keep on doing the same old thing every day. Experiencing an occasional lapse is expected and common, but many will end up shattering your desire for change entirely.

6. Find appropriate tools and adequate support for positive change. The process of changing a lifestyle may seem somewhat intimidating or disconcerting to many people because sustained habit change or new habit building requires breaking old and adopting new patterns of behavior. That is why getting any form of support or guidance while you undertake this challenge will encourage you to keep going.

A key element in any behavioral change is to surround yourself with people that have a positive influence on your life. Caring family members or friends often want what is best for you, and they are likely to support you in your struggles to become a better person. Stay away from anyone who interferes with your healthy choices or who tries to push you back to your old ways.

Partners or loved ones may help you create the right environment for change, overcome difficulties, or maintain commitment. And when you share your goals with other people, you allow them to make you accountable in tracking your progress. The more accountable you are to others, the more likely you are to stick to the initiative of achieving your goals.

Depending upon your circumstances, modifying some habitual behaviors may be more successful with the support of a coach or a medical professional. They can help you access valuable information and identify effective resources, or they can design an appropriate treatment for you.

You should consider exploring a wide variety of electronic tools created by experts to foster and sustain life changes. You can also access apps that help you increase your motivation and keep you on track. Some even penalize you for your lack of progress.

Finally, in my opinion, the process of getting rid of unhealthy behaviors is often packed with discouraging or negative connotations. Usually, too much emphasis is put either on the difficulty of the process or on the apparent high level of failure experienced by some people when making lifestyle changes. Those thoughts can make anyone afraid or reluctant to change.

As we modify our habits, our attention should be focused mostly on our resilience to overcome trials and on our limitless potential for improvement. Thus, locating and using various sources of inspiration on a regular basis will boost our positive thinking.

Read or watch inspirational materials about people who have accomplished something impressive despite their limitations or who have been able to thrive when they freed themselves from harmful habits. Allow yourself to be inspired by someone else's experiences and try to implement their recommendations into yours. Then, let your determination and motivation do the driving.

To keep in mind

- Knowledge and awareness can empower us in the process of making better life choices.

- You need to understand the reasons behind your urges so that you find appropriate ways to overcome them.

- Constructive opinions, advice, and feedback can be beneficial in the process of behavioral change.

- The challenge to change your behavior entails controlling the factors that favor or interfere with the expected results.

Questions to reflect on:

1. What role does your mind play in regulating your habits? Explain

2. Are most of your lifestyle choices controlled by your lower or higher brain?

3. What compelling reasons do you have to change undesirable habits?

4. Do you have any kind of support to rely on as you modify these behaviors?

Chapter 9:

Technology Detox for Better Mental Health

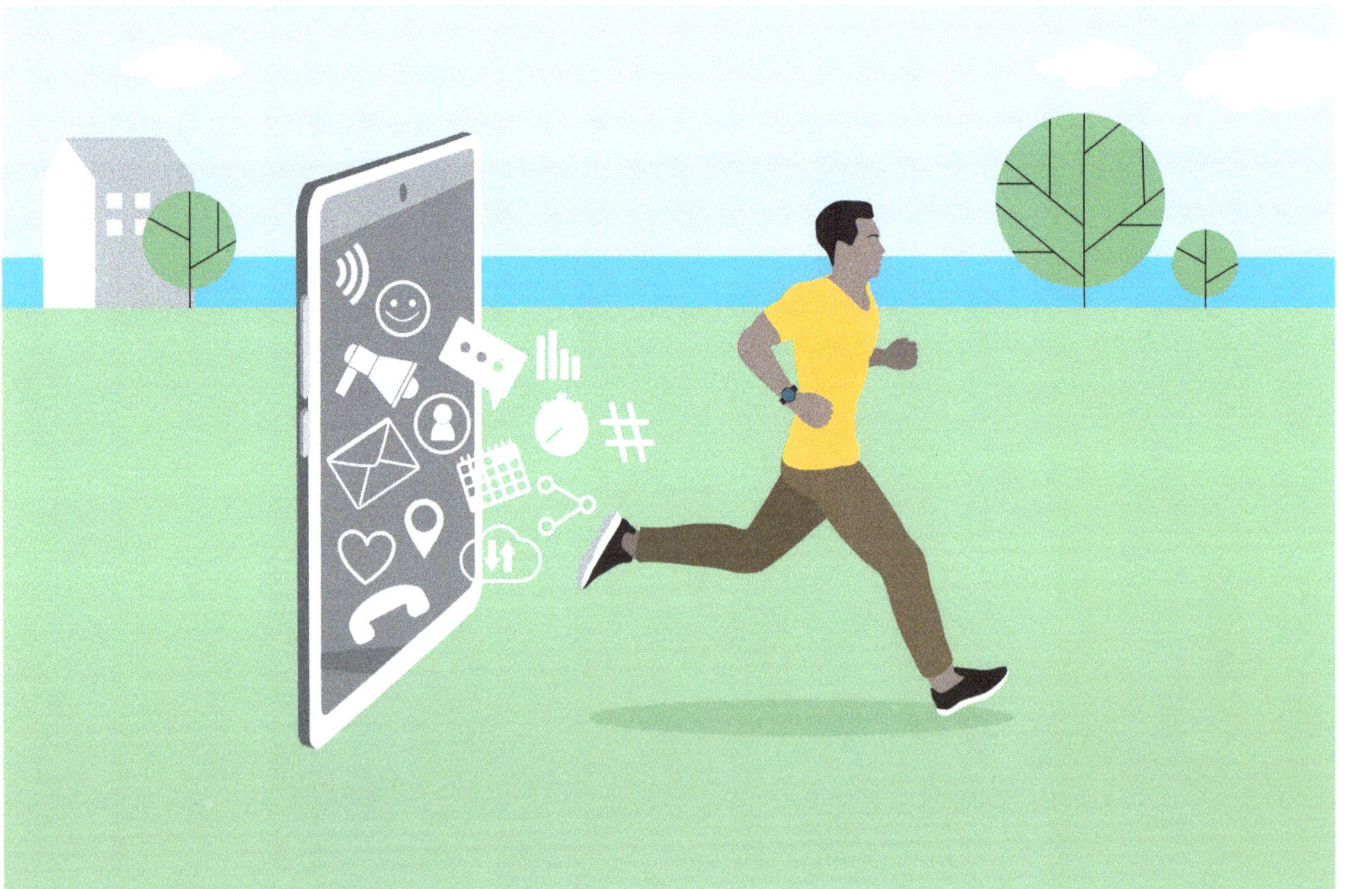

The impact of modern technology in our daily lives is immeasurable. This amazing human achievement encourages innovation, increases productivity, promotes creativity, and improves the quality of our lives. We all depend on the convenience of the digital world to accomplish most of our daily tasks because it offers great benefits like instant access to information and total connectivity. However, it also has disadvantages, including information overload, communication overburden, and intrusion on our privacy, among others. Furthermore, technology over-dependency can disconnect us from the real world and lead to addiction, thus preventing us from leading well-balanced lives.

Experts from different perspectives and disciplines have begun to make us aware of the unquestionably harmful impact that modern technology can have on our physical, mental, and emotional well-being. Many of us have somehow become enslaved by our devices, letting them control our actions, habits, and behaviors. Therefore, people who are unable to liberate themselves from the tight grip of their smartphones or computer screens suffer from psychological distress and behavioral problems at levels never seen before. To overcome the negative effects of misusing technology, we must take to heart its dangers and how it affects each of us on a personal level.

According to the experts, the excessive use of technology may increase stress levels, social isolation, physical inactivity, sleep deprivation, depression, and dementia. Unfortunately, about 70% of people between the ages of 25 and 35 in the United States are extremely dependent on their iPhones. They take them everywhere, using them from early morning to bedtime for work, school, entertainment, and shopping. Statistics indicate that the average American spends about seven hours staring at a screen and about two hours consuming social media. Unfortunately, technological and social media addiction is also becoming a pandemic worldwide.

Modern technology has changed our social environments, leading many people to feel moody, anxious, distracted, isolated, and exhausted. In addition, it has made some of us less capable of making wise decisions and less inclined to establish or maintain close personal relationships. However, technology is supposed to make our lives easier, not decrease our happiness or cause emotional suffering. Unfortunately, even though many people acknowledge that they have a problematic relationship with technology, they are unable to control their digital habits.

The first step to overcoming the adverse effects of digital compulsion is being able to differentiate the good uses of technology from the toxic ones. By developing an awareness of the various signs of digital overload, we can start setting personal boundaries, finding ways to make our devices less intrusive, or in other words, do a digital detox. Be aware of the following signs of techno addiction:

- Feeling an uncontrollable need to check your phone regularly
- Multitasking between devices throughout the day
- Being anxious or restless in the absence of your phone or device for more than a few minutes
- Neglecting responsibilities or not focusing on relevant tasks because you are immersed in using a device
- Feeling discomfort when interacting or socializing with people face-to-face
- Spending more time with virtual friends than with family or friends in person
- Browsing websites frequently to keep up with the latest news
- Spending too many hours scrolling on social media or playing video games and little or no time exercising or playing sports
- Having three or more social media accounts
- Feeling excessive preoccupation with social media updates, statuses, and likes
- Feeling the need to buy and use many electronic devices, software products, and digital games
- Having a loved one recommend you to reduce your screen time or phone usage

Given that technology and digital communication are here for the long term and that we can no longer function without our electronic devices, we must learn to navigate our virtual environments cautiously and find ways to prevent us from falling into excessive technological stimulation.

Being regularly exposed to digital overstimulation alters our brain chemistry and its balance. A hyperactive brain becomes restless and unable to unwind or relax. It can also make an individual crave more technological stimulation with an inability to stay away from digital gadgets. Eventually, this continual stress provokes emotional discomfort, exhaustion, and burnout. For this reason, we must not let digital over-dependency turn into a tech addiction.

Unlike humans, our devices do not have a living intelligence, the capacity to make the right choices for us, or the ability to use our time productively. Neither do they have feelings, emotions, or purposes in life. It is still up to each of us to determine how to act wisely. Overdependence on technological devices can lead to sacrificing our personal freedom allowing tech companies or others to lead our lives for us.

We must remember that there is more to life than reading text messages, watching viral videos, scrolling news or updates on social media, chatting, doing online shopping, or playing video games. The "real" world still offers a wide variety of gratifying experiences, enjoyable activities, and meaningful interactions to produce personal happiness and satisfaction.

Being a highly functioning person depends upon becoming an independent thinker, establishing meaningful relationships, developing a positive sense of self-worth, and crafting lives of meaning and purpose. Unfortunately, excessive-tech and social media consumption can lead us to become dysfunctional people.

Studies have found a correlation between frequent social media use and low or negative mood levels. Researchers have concluded that social media leads to stress and anxiety when we make our own decisions based on what others do, not on what we need or want. In addition, other people's actions and circumstances can alter our personal barometers compelling us to see ourselves through someone else's lenses. Obviously, living our lives according to other people's values and standards affects our emotional balance.

There are worthwhile benefits to putting aside our devices, especially if they interfere with our well-being and productivity. Choosing not to surrender to the unrestrained pleasures of our digital devices and or the slavery of public opinion have exceptional mental health results. To start, a digital detox can contribute to better attitudes, stronger relationships, and improved sleep quality.

A digital detox is oriented toward replacing problematic or unhealthy tech habits with healthy ones. It often requires that we take a break from all electronic devices or reduce screen time for a certain period of time. It may also include abstaining from using our phones, internet, TV streaming, social media, video games, chatting, etc. Usually, the time wasted with a digital gadget can be filled with rewarding activities that improve one's quality of life.

A tech detox can allow us to regain our autonomy and decision-making power. It can be achieved with a great deal of self-control to overcome our urge for instant gratification or with professional help and therapy if we are unable to curb our digital habits ourselves.

Steps to Consider in a Detox Plan

- Keep track of the time that you are spending online daily
- Analyze your tech habits and determine the behaviors that need to be kept under control or fully eliminated
- Identify the reasons why you need to modify these tech habits
- Make your own goals and create rules for your digital detox
- Determine how and when you will have tech-free time
- Commit to breaking the bad habit and making yourself accountable.
- Create positive routines to replace those you need to change
- Try to get out of the house to go to a gym, play a sport, or take a walk
- Assess and reward your progress regularly
- Use a digital detox app or a website blocker to regain control of your time.
- Block the internet temporarily using software like Self-control or Freedom
- Find a partner to support you along the way
- Avoid multitasking and use only one device at a time to prevent overstimulation.
- Don't use your phone while eating, driving, exercising, sleeping, or interacting with family and friends.

Breaking the cycle of digitally addictive behaviors is not easy for anyone. It involves acknowledging the problem and adopting positive life habits to improve your life. You can thrive in a technologically advanced world by making prudent, responsible, and mindful use of your devices without surrendering your will to them. Protecting your psychological health involves controlling your own habits so that they can carry you forward toward good health, inner harmony, and mental peace.

To keep in mind

- Technology over-dependency can disconnect you from the real world and lead to addiction, thus preventing you from leading a well-balanced life.

- Modern technology has changed social environments, making people feel moody, anxious, distracted, and isolated.

- Being regularly exposed to digital overstimulation alters your brain chemistry and its balance.

- The time wasted with a digital gadget can be filled with rewarding activities that improve your life quality.

Questions to reflect on:

1. Have you personally experienced any technology's disadvantages? Explain

2. Are you highly dependent on your electronic devices and have serious difficulties staying away from them?

3. From the list provided in this chapter, what signs of techno addiction do you have?

4. In what ways could reducing screen time improve the quality of your life?

5. Do you need a digital detox to curb your unhealthy tech habits? Would you need to rely on professional support?

Chapter 10:

Benefits of Spiritual and Religious Practices on Well-being

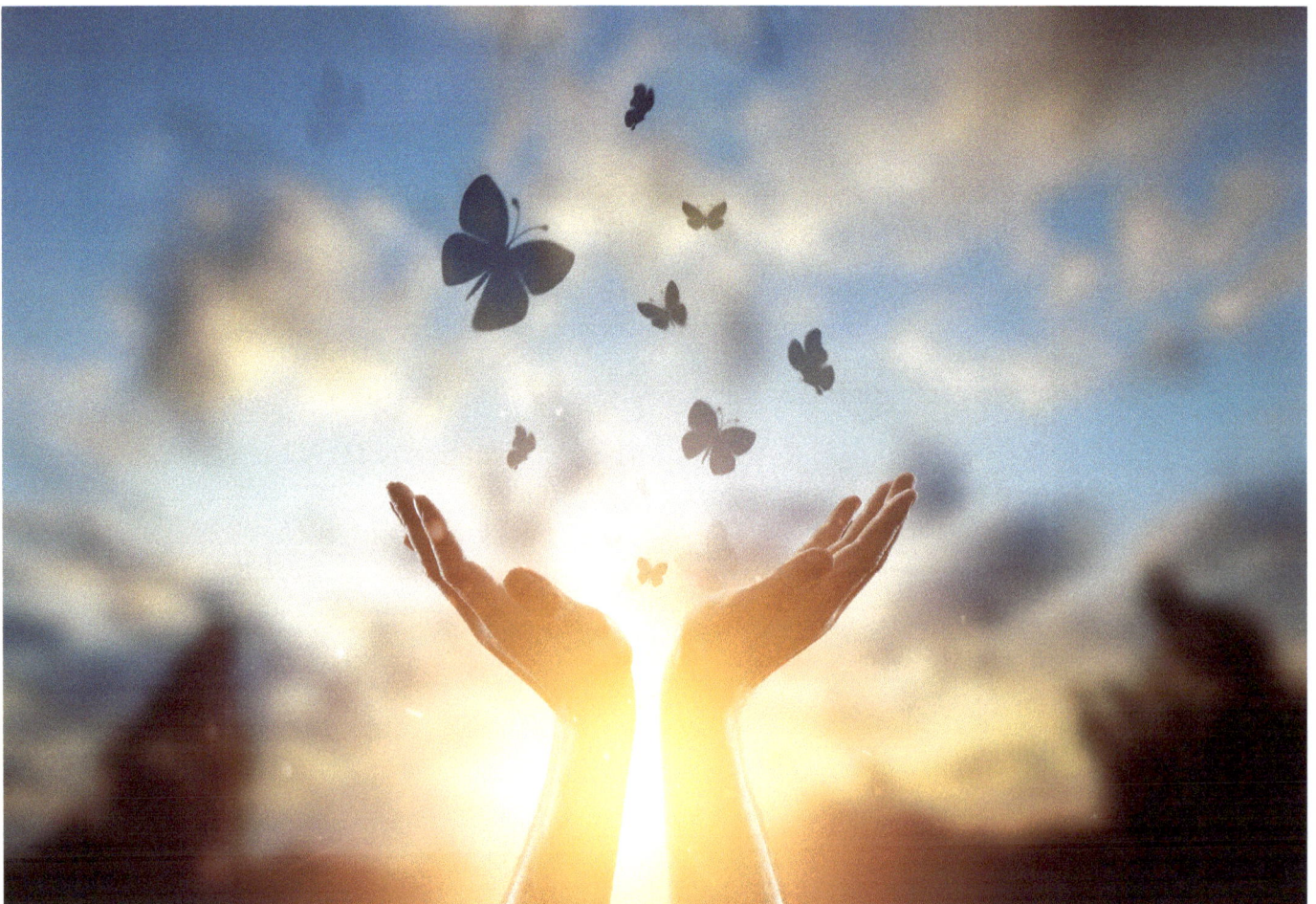

A vast majority of world cultures acknowledge the importance of integrating spiritual or religious activities into our daily lives to help us find the meaning and purpose of our existence, to cope better with adversity, and to bring peace and harmony to our minds. However, the secularization of modern societies has caused a decline in religious belief and participation, which coincides with a higher level of mental disorders, distress, and other negative outcomes among their populations.

Today, many people think that believing in God or having a genuine spiritual life is pointless and even irrational. Either they may not personally experience enough evidence of the existence of a higher power, or they expect science to give reasonable answers to the essential questions of life. Yet perhaps the essence of God cannot be appropriately understood with the logic and limitations of the human mind.

Currently, adolescents and young adults spend more time in their digital environments and little or no time in communities of faith. And even though about 75% of Millennials and Gen Z people consider themselves religious or spiritual, they are less likely to turn to God in times of uncertainty or crisis.

As more people disclose a lack of trust or commitment to organized religion, and perhaps even a passive indifference towards God, the unprecedented technological progress they enjoy has not become the source of happiness, fulfilment, and satisfaction they seek. Therefore, there are a lot of unhappy people in the world. The obvious questions one must ask are: What is missing in their lives? Are they having a severe spiritual crisis?

Developing spiritual or religious wisdom allows us to experience the mystery of the universe and marvel at the miracle of our existence. It also involves being aware of the realities of our physical and innermost being. It guides us in reflecting upon transcendental dilemmas such as origin, destiny, mortality, suffering, and injustice, and increases our capacity for understanding our world. It connects our intellectual concerns with our existential struggles. Spiritual and religious wisdom cause us to have an awareness of what really matters in life.

It should be stated that, even though the concepts of religion and spirituality may overlap, they sometimes follow different paths in their practice. While religion is a formal and organized system of beliefs accepted by a community of faith, spirituality is an individual mindset that connects with a sacred power beyond the self. Despite their differences, these two concepts are used here interchangeably.

In general, clinical science has been reluctant to establish a connection between religious or spiritual practices and our overall well-being. However, several recent scientific studies published in reputable medical journals have determined that religion is in fact a vital life-enhancing force with significant benefits for our body and mind. As a result, most medical facilities in the United States currently welcome the support of clergy or pastoral counselors for their patients.

Studies done at Duke University Medical Center, firmly documented in tangible data, show that people who are deeply religious experience better health and tend to live longer than those who are not. Furthermore, religious involvement appears to increase healing and survival even among severely ill people, thus providing a protective effect against mortality.

Research further indicates that people who are genuinely devout and attend church services regularly experience greater life satisfaction and happiness than those who are less active in their faith. Pious individuals experience additional benefits that include:

- Fewer negative emotional states and mental problems
- Lower levels of anxiety, depression, and suicide
- Less alcohol and drug abuse
- Fewer risk-taking behaviors
- Reduced levels of crime and delinquency
- Better coping and adaptation skills
- More positive attitudes toward life in general

It is important to note that, spiritual and religious beliefs can also be used in destructive and damaging ways. Practices associated with deviant religious groups, cults, or fundamentalists frequently contribute to discord, and foster intolerance, violence, and discrimination. Yet, irrational religious behaviors of some must not discourage others from cultivating a fertile spiritual life as a source of inner strength.

Contrary to what some people might believe, a reluctance to seek God can result in personal dissatisfaction, hopelessness, and suffering in the world. It also causes us to forget that true happiness comes from within ourselves and not from what happens to us or the circumstances of our lives.

A strong faith is not only one of the most effective healing resources available to us, but also a source of inspiration and positive emotions such as gratitude, comfort, and peace, among others. Furthermore, belonging to close-knit religious or spiritual groups allows people to share their burdens, avoid isolation, and receive community support in challenging times.

Humans long for a spiritual connection with a higher power to overcome uncertainty and provide direction to their lives. In fact, most faith communities focus on the importance of building a trusting relationship with God to experience His love, provision, and guidance. They also present God as the perfect intelligence who loves us and is the source of all goodness.

Most religions use various tools to facilitate the spiritual growth of their followers and plant the seeds of a conscious awareness of God. Prayer, meditation, contemplation, and mindfulness are joyful experiences that bring spiritual restoration to our hearts and minds. They change our vision of the world and silence the noise of our fears, concerns, and frustrations. Ah, and they radically transform the way we think about our problems.

Religious and spiritual practices remind us that our lives serve greater purposes and that we need to move beyond ourselves to enhance the lives of others around us. They promote values like kindness, forgiveness, and compassion oriented to foster harmony. They encourage us to share our talents and abilities to create a better world. And by helping others and developing caring relationships, we boost our own mental and emotional health.

On a personal level, I can say that prayer has changed the direction of my life, and that it has filled it with an enduring joy. I fully rely on the power of prayer to overcome a variety of challenges because it helps me stay grounded in stressful times, or simply when my well gets a bit dry. Having a strong faith makes me more patient and increases my capacity to endure the various challenges life brings my way. It is the best medicine for my burdened heart.

Prayer gives me an inner wisdom and a positive mindset, preventing me from feeling helpless or discouraged. It makes me more appreciative of the countless blessings bestowed on me, liberating my mind from the prison of victimhood. I am certain that the daily practice of prayer can lead anyone to an effective mental and emotional rejuvenation, and that through this means anyone can embrace God's divinity.

Every morning I sit down for a moment of prayer and spiritual reflection to let God guide my actions, awaken my gratitude, and bring the best out in me. As I prepare myself to face the new day, I open my heart to Him, inviting Him into my life. And each time I seek His presence, I feel more connected with Him. This loving relationship fills my heart with a profound serenity.

Personal crisis can lead us to reexamine our views about God and redirect our attention to our faith. Setbacks also remind us that our neglected soul is an essential part of our humanity. And just as our body needs to be sustained with food, our spirit must be nourished with comfort-seeking, faith-based experiences to increase our well-being.

Building an authentic religious life is a journey that begins with seeking God's presence in your life and making it a priority. This goal is achieved through various means that include constant prayer, collective worship, spiritual activities, and inspirational readings. As you advance along your path, you will soon discover that a complete trust in God is the most effective instrument to navigate the choppy waters of this world. It can help you emerge from the darkness of any ordeal with the capacity to appreciate the extraordinary fortune of being alive and even revel in the outlook of an everlasting life.

- Developing spiritual or religious wisdom allows us to experience the mystery of the universe and marvel at the miracle of our existence.

- Scientific studies show that people who are deeply religious experience better health and live longer than those who are not.

- A strong faith is one of the most effective healing resources available, bringing restoration to hearts and minds.

- Building a strong spiritual or religious life can be achieved through meditation, prayer, collective worship, and inspirational readings.

Questions to reflect on:

1. What is the state of your spiritual and/or religious life at the moment? Explain

2. Could becoming a more spiritual or religious person make you experience greater satisfaction in life?

3. What benefits would such a change bring to your emotional and mental health?

4. Have you had any personal crisis in the past that made you reexamine your relationship with God or a Higher power?

Chapter 11:

Relaxation: Relieving Stress Naturally and Effectively

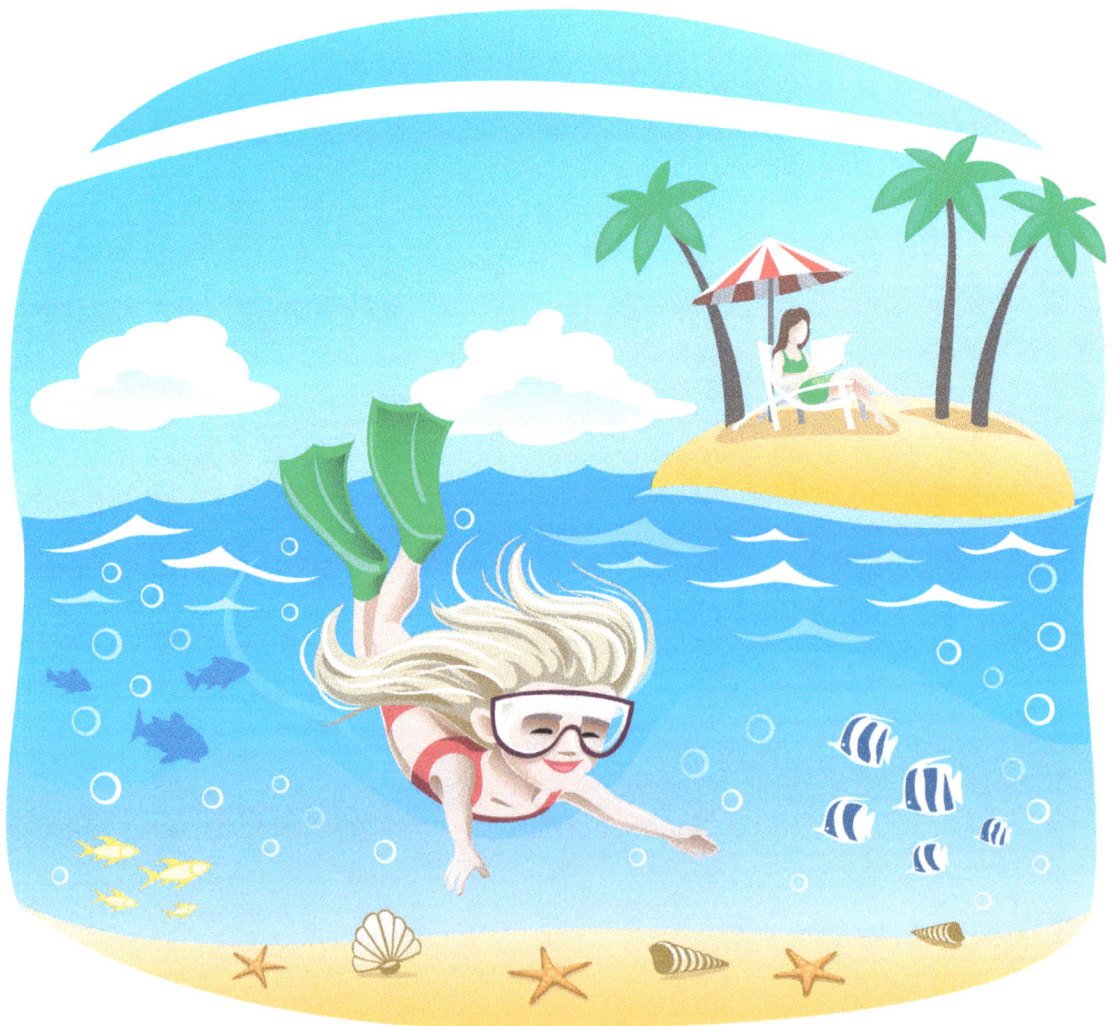

Most of us live in a fast-paced, noisy world which deprives us of opportunities to liberate ourselves from multiple stressors. The futility of so many distractions take up our time, filling our minds with anxious thoughts and all sorts of pressures. They keep us in a permanent agitated state where silence and tranquility usually disappear. As a result, some people adopt unhealthy stress-managing practices such as binge drinking, drugs, smoking, and overeating as stress relievers.

Instead, there are hundreds of feel-good activities available to increase our general well-being. These positive resources allow us to intentionally reduce the permanent siege of our electronic devices, walk away from the haste of our daily lives, and create healing spaces to regain our mental balance and inner peace.

Here are some natural remedies to reduce stress:

1. Practicing deep breathing for wellness. Breathing provides oxygen which increases high-energy chemicals in our body. In addition, the deliberate process of taking slow and deep breaths helps people unwind from stress and anxiety in a dramatic way. Since stress plays an important role in the development of various diseases, the use of breathing techniques can break the patterns of tension we often encounter.

The therapeutic effects of rhythmic conscious breathing are immediately evident to those who practice it regularly; they are also acknowledged by the medical community. Deep breathing reduces heart rate and blood pressure, improves mood, reduces pain, and improves performance. The ultimate effect of breathing is inner peace, which is feeling relaxed and balanced.

There are different breathing techniques that you can use for relaxation. Here are some examples:

The Sequence Of 4-7-8 Breathing

— Sit in a comfortable position with your eyes closed

— Inhale through your nose as you silently count to 4

— Hold your breath as you silently count to 7

— Exhale through your mouth as you silently count to 8

— Repeat this breathing pattern at least five more times

The Belly Breathing

— Sit or lie flat in a comfortable position with your eyes closed

— Place one hand on your belly and the other on your chest

— Inhale deeply through your nose and belly

— Let your belly push your hand in

— Slowly breathe out through your pursed lips

— Use the hand in your belly to push all air out

— Repeat this technique at least 8 more times

The Alternate Nostril Breath

— Sit in a comfortable position with your eyes closed

— Lift your right hand toward your nose

— Exhale completely and use your right thumb to close your right nostril

— Inhale through your left nostril and then close the left nostril with your finger

— Open the right nostril and exhale through this side

— Inhale through your right nostril and close the right nostril with your finger

— Open the left nostril and exhale through this side

— This completes one cycle

— Repeat the cycle for five or ten minutes

2. Doing meditation. This practice has been recognized as an essential path to mental wellness and longevity. A main goal of meditation is to remove chaotic thoughts from our mind and replace them with a sense of calm and a mindfulness of the present moment. It connects mind, body, and spirit, allowing us to disconnect ourselves from external stimuli and to focus on our inner compass instead.

Meditation is known for relieving stress and anxiety by making us pause in the midst of turmoil, developing acceptance of difficult emotions, and promoting inner harmony. And even though it is often associated with religious and spiritual development, it can be practiced by anyone regardless of their beliefs.

There are various types of meditation practices to choose from. Explore some of them online through free and paid websites and apps. Identify the one that best meets your needs.

Types of Meditation Practices	
Mindfulness	Transcendental
Spiritual	Progressive
Focused	Loving-kindness
Mantra	Visualization

Meditation has become very popular worldwide among people who experience its great benefits. It has been suggested that 30 minutes of daily meditation may alleviate mild anxiety symptoms and act as an antidepressant. Beginners can try 5-to-10-minute sessions.

To get started, you should commit to a style of meditation and practice it regularly until it becomes comfortable and enjoyable. The regular practice of meditation is believed to lead to experiencing true happiness. Additional meditation benefits include:

Meditation benefits

- Improved concentration and cognitive ability
- Reduced aggression and angry outbursts
- Improved emotional regulation
- Greater patience, tolerance, and empathy toward others
- Controlled impulses and addictive behaviors
- Increased willpower and self-discipline
- Improved sleep habits and sleep quality
- Increased pain tolerance
- Improved immunity and healthy aging
- Enhanced mood and positive thinking
- Decreased stress, anxiety, and depression

3. Communicating feelings to others. As children, we are trained to express good emotions and repress uncomfortable feelings such as anger, sadness, frustration, and fear. But emotions are neither good nor bad. They are instinctive responses to experiences and life events. Thus, acknowledging our feelings and being understood by others are basic human needs.

Many people feel embarrassed or afraid to share their feelings with loved ones, peers, and colleagues. They may not want to appear vulnerable, be judged, or be ignored. Yet, masking our feelings until they start to hurt us can lead to exhaustion, meltdowns, or illness. In contrast, talking about our concerns with our support network helps us identify and validate our emotions.

Receiving emotional support can make a big difference in the way we cope with our problems or feelings, especially when we seem unable to handle a personal crisis. Discussing our emotions with someone we trust, a therapist, or a group can help us gain a new perspective to move forward. It can also lead to releasing tension and lifting a heavy weight off our shoulders.

Furthermore, voicing our inner thoughts and emotions helps us to connect with others in meaningful ways. Effective communication is vital to establishing and maintaining strong relationships. In healthy relationships, people must be mutually receptive to each other's needs and feelings and be willing to engage in open and honest dialogue as often as possible.

Although successful communication is not always guaranteed, it is your responsibility to find adequate ways to express your feelings. The following recommendations will facilitate this process:

- Avoid heated arguments in moments of disagreements
- Take time to analyze your emotions before discussing them with others
- Find an adequate opportunity to convey your feelings to someone else
- If possible, plan the conversation ahead of time
- Make sure you have the other person's attention
- Remain calm and choose a non-confrontational approach
- Be honest and direct but pay attention to your body language
- Make an effort to be an attentive listener
- If face-to-face dialogue becomes difficult, express your emotions in writing

4. Listening, playing, and composing music. The therapeutic power of music to improve overall mental health has been acknowledged in the medical world for many years. Music has become a healing tool to treat mental and physical ailments in hospitals, rehabilitation centers, schools, nursing homes, and hospices.

Listening, playing, and composing music are pleasurable activities that trigger positive responses in the brain. They release feel-good hormones like dopamine and endorphins. Some types of music can be soothing or relaxing, while others can be energizing and invigorating. There is no doubt that music is an effective mood enhancer and a stress distractor because it entertains and calms our minds.

Singing and dancing draw our thoughts away from concerns, worries, and problems. They reduce mental distress and rumination, calm our nervous system, and lower our heart rate. Furthermore, when we enjoy music with other people, we reinforce our social connections and overcome feelings of isolation.

5. Aromatherapy and Essential Oils. Although research on the effectiveness of essential oils on our health is limited, aromatherapy has become a well-known form of alternative medicine to aid in healing and recovery. Aromatherapy uses fragrant essential oils from plants to enhance both physical and emotional well-being. Stress, fear, or worry have a negative impact on our mental health and our immune system, reducing the body's capacity to fight infection and disease.

Essential oils are thought to stimulate smell receptors in the nose and trigger high emotional responses. They also contribute to relaxing the nervous system. These natural and gentle remedies may be inhaled directly or added to a warm bath or diffuser. They can also be applied to the skin, and as they travel through the bloodstream, they are believed to promote whole-body healing.

Multiple benefits have been associated with aromatherapy. Inhaled aroma from essential oils can boost cognitive performance, strengthen the immune system, provide natural pain relief, reduce inflammation, enhance mood, and induce sleep.

Stress Relief

Lavender, Bergamot, Chamomile, Lemon, Orange, Patchouli, Vanilla.

Anxiety/Fear

Frankincense, Jasmine, Lavender, Bergamot, Chamomile (Roman), Cedarwood, Neroli, Patchouli, Rose, Sandalwood.

Sadness/Grief

Sage, Bergamot, Chamomile (Roman), Clary Frankincense, Grapefruit, Jasmine, Lavender, Mandarin, Lemon, Orange, Rose, Sandalwood.

Immune system

Eucalyptus, Clove, Lavender, Tea tree, Oregano, Frankincense

6. Yoga. The word yoga means "union" and refers to a discipline that originated in India. It combines meditation, breathing techniques, and physical postures to connect the body, mind, and spirit. Although yoga started as a religious practice, it has become very popular in promoting higher levels of physical and mental well-being. Yoga is highly recommended for body relaxation and stress management.

The most common form of yoga practiced in the Western world is Hatha yoga, but there are other yoga styles. Some forms include gentle movements, while others require physically demanding ones. According to experts, any form of yoga offers many benefits, such as increased serenity and peace of mind, trimmer and better-toned bodies, improved balance, and greater flexibility.

The safest way to undertake yoga is by participating in a beginner's course with a trained instructor in a studio, a gym, or online. An instructor will help you become familiar with the various poses, provide tips to prevent injuries, guide you through proper breathing, and focus your attention on aligning your body and mind. In yoga, repetition, and consistency are important to gain confidence and achieve progress. For best results, aim to practice it two or three times a week.

7. Exercise. Get moving to manage stress and boost serotonin and endorphins. Exercise is one of the easiest ways to decrease stress levels and distract our minds from daily worries and frustrations. Any form of exercise, whether it is aerobics, walking, or practicing a sport, can be used to relieve stress.

Movement alters our state of consciousness and allows our concerns to take a back seat. It is an ideal mental booster. After an outdoor walk, a nature hike, several laps in a pool, or a racquetball game, for instance, we improve our ability to solve problems and regulate our emotions. Therefore, physical activity should become an important part of a stress management plan. Any form of physical activity helps us unwind and regain control over our emotions, bodies, and life.

8. Reading, gardening, and board games. These are additional tools that can help alleviate stress. Reading is an educational, relaxing, and enjoyable activity that provides mental stimulation and reduces mental decline. People who read regularly show lower levels of stress and depression than non-readers. Its positive effects are like those of meditation.

To get the recreational benefits derived from reading, you must put away your phone for at least 30 minutes and go over enjoyable materials in a quiet place, free from interruptions. Reading about someone else's experiences can be both enriching and inspiring. It can also help you gain wisdom as you face challenging situations or at least forget about your own worries temporarily.

Gardening is a mood-enhancing practice that gives many people a great deal of pleasure and joy. Planting trees, taking care of plants, and creating beautiful gardens offer opportunities to enjoy the sunlight, breathe fresh air, spend time outdoors, connect with nature, and get a full body workout. In addition, a garden can be a sanctuary to relax, unwind and meditate.

Getting started with gardening might seem a bit daunting; however, you can experiment by learning to take care of a few plants. Do not get discouraged if they die. This happens even to experienced gardeners. Find plants that require little care on your part until you become more skilled. Get information and tips from friends, neighbors, or in books and magazines. You can also join a garden club.

Board games have been a popular form of entertainment throughout history. They offer enormous mental and emotional benefits to people of all ages. To start, reducing time spent on electronic devices opens opportunities for anyone to have face-to-face interactions and strengthen bonds with family and friends. There is a great variety of games that can be played anywhere and anytime.

Playing board games contributes to stress release by distracting the mind from difficult emotions. When we have a good time, we feel more cheerful and content as our mind detaches from our troubles. Board games bring people closer through fun and laughter, which decrease cortisol levels and increase endorphins. Socializing and establishing connections is an effective way to create happiness.

Board games are also an excellent practice to increase mental agility and protect cognitive health. Some games require attention to detail and the use of critical skills such as memory, logic, problem-solving, and strategic thinking. There is no doubt that playing casual games is good for maintaining mental balance, sharp thinking, and joy.

To keep in mind

- Deep breathing reduces heart rate and blood pressure, improves mood, reduces pain, and improves performance.

- Meditation can relieve stress and anxiety by replacing chaotic thoughts with a sense of calm and peace.

- Listening, playing, and composing music has therapeutic effects such as relaxation and stress reduction.

- Reading is an educational, relaxing, and enjoyable activity that provides mental stimulation and reduces mental decline.

- Board games are entertaining and offer enormous mental and emotional benefits to people of all ages.

Questions to reflect on:

1. Have you ever experienced the soothing effects of meditation? How did it help you?

2. Do you usually share your concerns and feelings with family or friends or do you usually prefer not to talk about them with anyone?

3. How often do you read for relaxation or inspiration? Should you do it more frequently?

Chapter 12:

Must-Have Preventive Medical Tests and Screenings for Adults

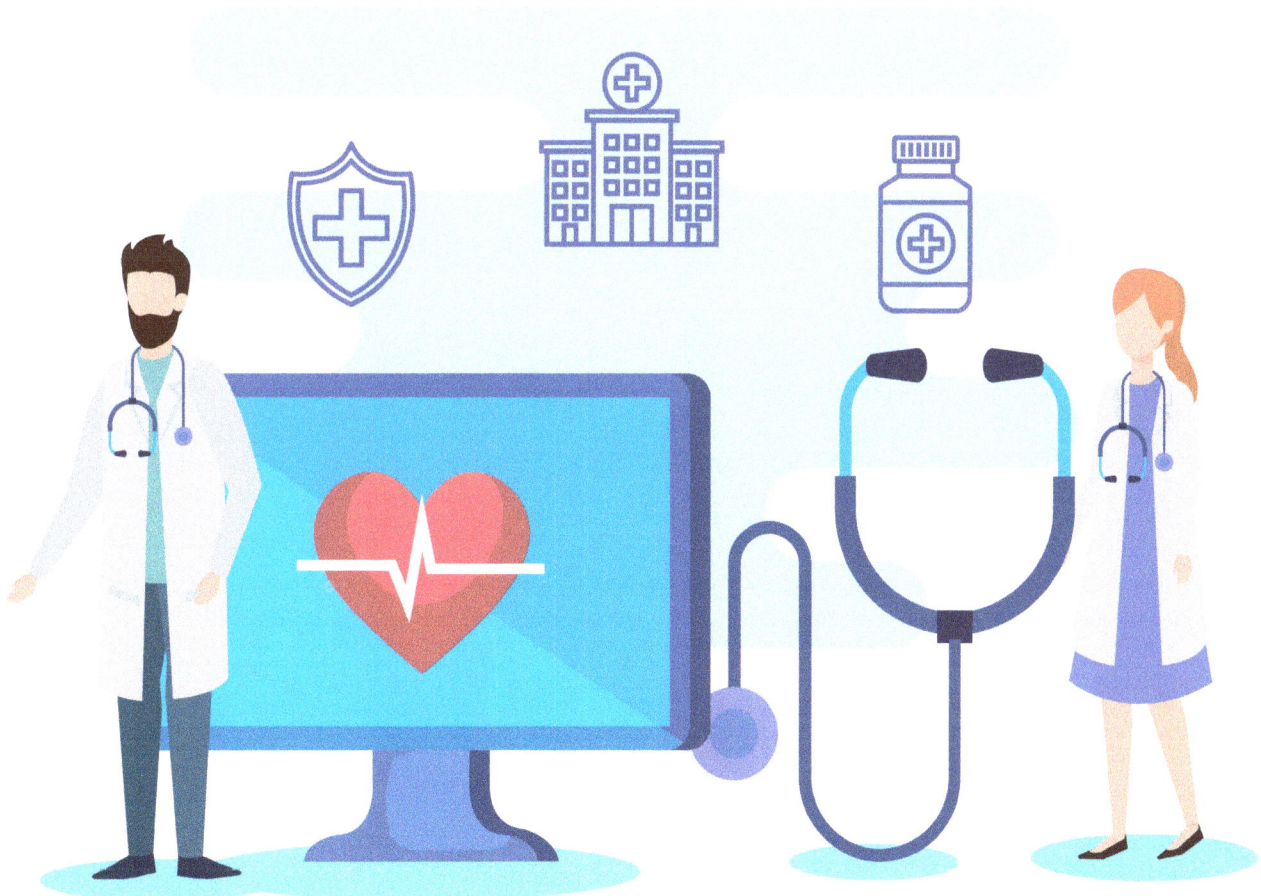

Consulting a doctor for regular checkups is a crucial step in taking responsibility for your well-being. Your physician will determine the appropriate timing and frequency of your medical tests based on your age, overall health, and your family's medical history. Prevention is more convenient, less painful, and less expensive than finding a cure for any ailment.

Preventive medical screenings help doctors assess your health status and the condition of your organs, allowing them to identify your potential risks for developing chronic diseases. The goal of early detection is usually making lifestyle changes, maintaining surveillance to reduce the risk of disease, or treating the first symptoms effectively.

Here are the most common tests ordered by doctors:

1. High-Cholesterol test. Cholesterol screening is performed by a blood test. All adults age 20 or older should have their cholesterol checked every four years, or more often, if certain factors put you at higher risk. Cholesterol is a waxy substance that can be found in all parts of the body, especially veins and arteries. It is produced by the liver from meat, poultry, and dairy products.

Foods high in saturated and trans-fats cause the liver to produce cholesterol in excess, which becomes unhealthy. High cholesterol in your blood represents a risk to your health. It causes cardiovascular diseases such as heart disease and stroke. According to cardiologists, about 80% of heart disease and stroke are preventable. That is why you must be aware of your cholesterol levels.

There are two types of cholesterol: **LDL** cholesterol, which is bad, and **HDL**, which is good. High LDL levels will build up in the inner walls of the arteries that feed the heart and brain. Along with high LDL levels, additional risk factors for coronary disease include obesity, physical inactivity, and diabetes. When it comes to cholesterol:

- **Check** your numbers and assess your risk.
- **Change** your diet and lifestyle to help improve your levels.
- **Control** your cholesterol with help from your doctor if needed.

Below is a general cholesterol levels guideline:

Cholesterol Levels Guideline			
	Desirable	**Border High**	**High**
Total Cholesterol	Less than **200**	**200 - 239**	**240** and higher
LDL Cholesterol	Less than **130**	**130 - 159**	**160** and higher
HDL Cholesterol	**50** and higher	**40 - 49**	Less than **40**
Triglycerides	Less than **200**	**200 - 399**	**400** and higher

2. Blood pressure test. All adults, starting at 18, should have their blood pressure measured at regular checkups or with a home device. Blood pressure is a good indicator of your overall health. High blood pressure is one of the most common cardiovascular problems. It affects the body's arteries and major organs, such as the heart, the kidneys, and the eyes.

High blood pressure, also called hypertension, puts people at high risk of life-threatening conditions. It is considered a "silent killer" because of its lack of symptoms, which may include headaches, nosebleeds, and shortness of breath.

When the force of the blood pushing through the vessels is consistently high, the heart must work harder to pump blood. The more blood the heart has to pump through narrower arteries, the higher the blood pressure gets. If left untreated, hypertension can damage blood vessels and lead to heart and kidney failure, vision loss, and sexual dysfunction.

High blood pressure is associated with various risk factors that include age, family history, overweight, obesity, lack of exercise, tobacco use, excessive salt intake and low potassium levels, stress, and high alcohol consumption. Here is a blood pressure level chart.

Blood Pressure Levels			
Blood pressure category	Systolic mm Hg (upper #)		**Diastolic mm Hg (lower #)**
Low	**Less than 90**	and	**Less than 60**
Normal	**Less than 120**	and	**Less than 80**
Elevated	**120 - 129**	and	**Less than 80**
High (Hypertension Stage 1)	130 - 139	or	80 - 89
High (Hypertension Stage 2)	**140 or higher**	or	**90 or higher**
Hypertensive crisis (Seek emergency care)	**Higher than 180**	and/or	Higher than 120

3. Diabetes risk test. Measures your blood glucose or sugar levels to determine if they are normal or abnormal. The test can be done after fasting or at random during the day. A glucose and diabetes test is recommended for all adults starting at age 45, for individuals with a family history of diabetes, or if you are overweight or obese, given that people in these groups are more likely to develop this disorder.

When you eat carbohydrates, your body turns them into glucose to be used as energy. Having too much or too little glucose in your blood might indicate a serious medical disorder. Diabetes causes your blood levels to rise.

If left untreated, chronically elevated levels of blood sugar can lead to even more serious conditions, including kidney disease, heart failure, and blindness. If diagnosed at an early stage, adequate precautions will be taken before complications develop. Use the following chart as a guideline:

Blood Glucose Chart			
Mg / DL	**Fasting**	**After Eating**	2 – 3 hours After Eating
Normal	**80 - 100**	**170 - 200**	120 - 140
Impaired Glucose	**101 - 125**	**190 - 230**	140 - 160
Diabetic	**126 +**	**220 - 300**	200 plus

4. Colonoscopy. This test is used to investigate gastrointestinal issues and to check for signs of colorectal cancer. This is a very common type of cancer, and if caught early, it can be treated in about 90% of people. Early detection can improve treatment outcomes. If undetected, colon cancer can spread to other tissues or organs.

Health organizations recommend screening for colon cancer or colon polyps at age 50 or earlier if you have a family history or other risk factors. During this screening, a tiny video camera is used by a doctor to view the inside of the entire colon and rectum to look for changes, irritations, polyps (small growths), or cancer. If necessary, polyps and abnormal tissue are removed.

5. Mammogram. It is a breast X-ray picture to detect changes in breast tissue that could be cancerous. Regular mammograms reduce breast cancer mortality significantly and make early treatment less invasive. An abnormal mammogram does not always indicate the presence of cancer. In such a case, additional follow-up screenings will be required.

Although medical experts do not seem to agree on when and how often women should get a mammogram, many consider that women should get a yearly mammogram at age 40 or earlier if there are risk factors involved. Women 55 or older can have mammograms every two years if the previous tests have been normal.

Mammograms work best when their results can be compared with previous breast screenings. This allows radiologists to identify changes. In any case, your doctor can guide you based on your family history or individual concerns. Women with close relatives who have had breast cancer are considered at high risk.

Along with mammograms, women are advised to do regular breast examinations to detect abnormal changes such as lumps, pain, unusual skin appearance or nipple discharge.

6. Pap Smear test or Papanicolaou. It is a women's diagnostic test for abnormal cell development around the cervix that could turn into cancer. It is an important tool in women's health. It involves collecting sample cells from your cervix that will be sent to a lab and a pelvic examination of the vagina, uterus, and rectum.

Women 21 to 65 should get a Pap smear every three years, or more often if there are abnormal results. If the results indicate cancerous or precancerous cells, your physician will require further tests and treatment.

Although cervical cancer is most common in women over age 40, your doctor will decide when you should begin Pap testing based on your risk factors. Cervical cancer is a progressive disease; therefore, early detection is crucial. If not treated, it could spread to nearby lymph glands and into the uterus.

7. Prostate Cancer test. Prostate cancer is perhaps the most common cancer among men older than 50, yet it rarely causes any symptoms before that age. Early prostate cancer may be discovered by rectal examination in a physical checkup, an enlarged prostate, or a blood test called Prostate-specific antigen or PSA.

PSA is a blood test that measures the prostate-specific antigen levels in the blood. Antigens are substances that provoke responses from a person's immune system. The prostate-specific antigen levels can be elevated in the presence of prostate cancer.

Screening for elevated PSA levels beginning at age 55 helps reduce the risk of prostate cancer. The PSA level in blood is measured in units called nanograms per milliliter (ng/mL). The chance of having prostate cancer increases as the PSA level goes up, but there is no specific set cutoff point that can tell, without a doubt, if a man does or doesn't have prostate cancer.

Many doctors use a PSA cutoff point of 4 ng/mL or higher when deciding if an individual might need further testing, while others might recommend it starting at a lower level, such as 2.5 or 3. That is because a level below 4 does not guarantee the absence of cancer completely. Men with a PSA between 4 and 10 (called a borderline range) have about a 25% chance of having cancer. If the PSA is higher than 10, the chance of having cancer is over 50%.

If cancer is suspected, a prostate biopsy is often required. However, you must discuss your options with your doctor to help you choose any additional testing you are comfortable with and any potential treatment according to your age and family history.

8. Vision and hearing and tests. Sight and hearing screenings help care professionals detect problems with these important sensory organs before they fully develop and while they are most treatable. Children and adults should have their eyes and ears examined regularly depending on age and potential risks.

Activities with computers, smartphones, and video games can affect eyes and ears to a greater extent if improperly used. Screen lights, loud music, and noises can cause eye disorders and hearing loss. Also, wearing blue light glasses and sunglasses that protect your eyes from UV light is highly recommended.

Adults with no symptoms of eye or ear problems should have a comprehensive diagnostic evaluation of their eyes and ears at age 40 to prevent age-related hearing and vision loss. About 60% of adults will start experiencing some degree of vision and hearing loss by age 60. Therefore, eyes and ears should be checked every two to five years.

9. Dental screening. It is a checkup of your teeth, gums, and mouth tissues done by a dentist. It is used to detect cavities, tooth decay, gum disease, and other oral health problems early. It may include a comprehensive mouth evaluation combined with x-rays and other diagnostic tests.

Dental problems can become serious, painful, and expensive if not treated on time. Think of every tooth as a priceless jewel that you must care for and protect. People with gum disease may need more frequent examinations and treatment to avoid infection and tooth loss.

Most children and all adults should get a comprehensive dental exam periodically and a dental cleaning every six months. Checkups are also used to educate people on the best ways to care for their teeth and maintain good oral habits.

Good oral habits for everyone include:

- Brushing your teeth twice a day (for about two minutes each time)
- Using toothpaste that has fluoride
- Flossing at least once a day to remove food particles
- Replacing your toothbrush every three months
- Eating a healthy diet, avoiding sweets and sugary drinks
- Not smoking

- Regular medical tests and screenings are crucial for the early detection of various chronic disease risks.

- Keeping cholesterol and blood pressure levels under control help prevent cardiovascular disorders.

- Diabetes can lead to serious medical conditions including kidney disease, heart failure and blindness.

- Regular mammograms and pap smears reduce cancer mortality significantly and make early treatment less invasive.

- Children and adults should have regular dental, vision, and hearing screenings to detect early problems.

Questions to reflect on:

1. Do you regularly take common, preventive medical tests to assess the condition of your health?

2. Are you aware of your current cholesterol, blood pressure, and glucose levels?

3. Have you ever taken any screening for cancer prevention?

4. When was the last time you had:

    - A vision screening?

    - A hearing test?

    - A dental checkup?

Chapter 13:

Preventable Chronic Disorders and Diseases

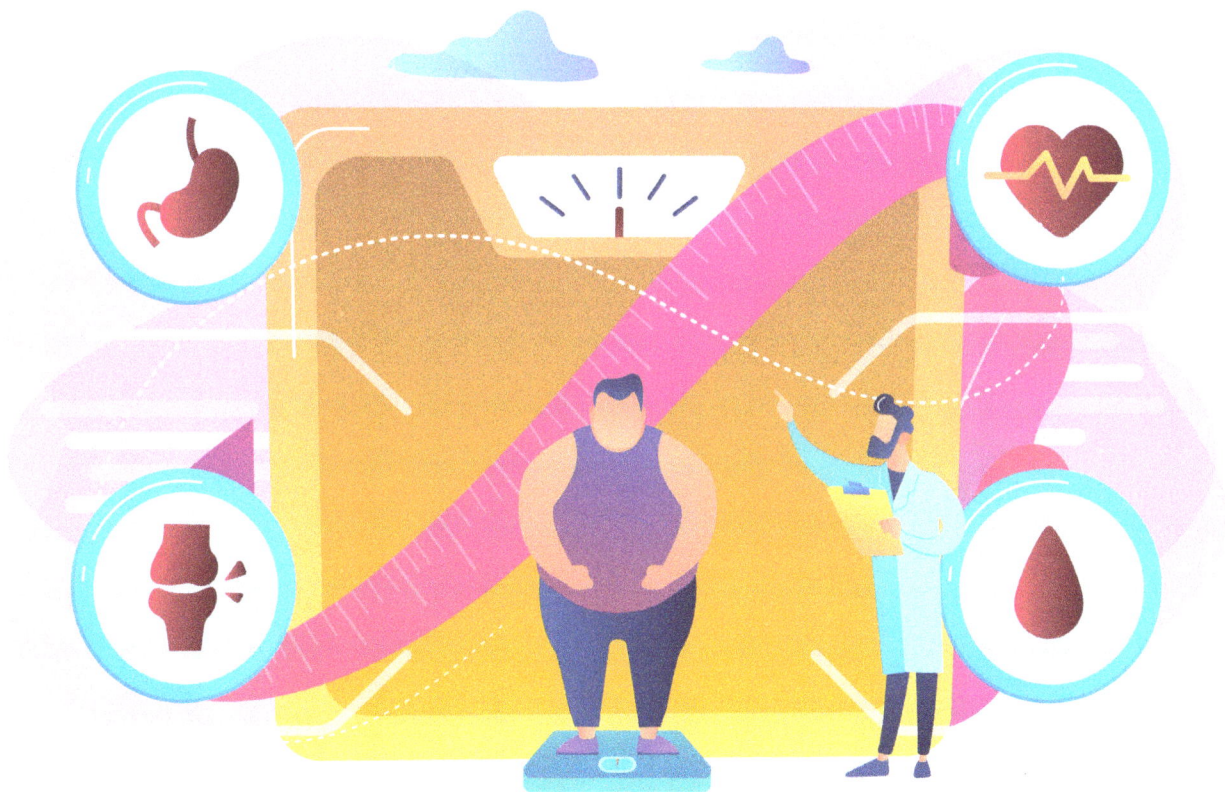

As it has been pointed out throughout this book, many chronic diseases are caused by poor habits and risky behaviors. Thus, anyone who learns to make healthy choices early in life can prevent developing many chronic ailments.

Chronic sicknesses, including heart disease, stroke, diabetes, and cancer, are the most common health problems in the United States, causing about 70% of deaths and, in other cases, leading to early disability. Furthermore, among adults ages 20 to 75, diabetes is the leading cause of kidney failure, blindness, and lower extremity amputations.

It is never too late to adopt habits that reduce the devastating consequences of chronic diseases. Evidently, the best way to control any chronic disease is prevention rather than getting medical treatment.

The most common risk factors for chronic diseases are:

Smoking	Excessive alcohol consumption
High blood pressure	Lack of regular medical checkups
High cholesterol	Not getting recommended screenings
Obesity	Family history
Physical inactivity	Other diseases like diabetes

Coronary heart disease: A heart attack happens when the blood flowing to the heart is significantly reduced or blocked. A blockage often results from a buildup of fat and cholesterol. The body attempts to repair the problem by generating tissue that thickens the vessel wall. As more fat and cholesterol accumulate, the vessel flow is further constricted.

Sometimes a plaque can rupture and form a clot that blocks the blood flow completely. A lack of blood flow can destroy part of the heart tissue. The damaged tissue or muscle cannot be repaired or reversed.

Although heart attacks are considered the biggest killer of middle age and older people in the United States and other developed countries, research indicates that this disease begins to develop in the teen years in many cases.

Unfortunately, a person rarely experiences any symptoms until the disease is way advanced. Some individuals may have mild warning signs, like chest pain that does not go away, which they often disregard. But it can also happen that an attack strikes suddenly, and a person dies even before any symptoms appear.

Common heart attack symptoms may include:

- Chest pain that may feel like pressure, tightness, or aching
- Pain or discomfort that spreads to the shoulder, arm, back, neck, or the upper belly
- Lightheadedness or dizziness
- Nausea
- Shortness of breath
- Heartburn or indigestion
- Cold sweat
- Fatigue

A heart attack is a life-threatening emergency that requires immediate medical attention. The sooner a person gets help the better the chance of a successful recovery.

Stroke: A brain attack that happens when a clot blocks an artery that feeds part of the brain (thrombosis or embolism) or when a portion of the artery or a blood vessel bursts, causing a cerebral hemorrhage. As a result, the injured area can be partially or permanently damaged, impairing the mental and physical functioning controlled by the affected side of the brain.

Common stroke symptoms include:

- Difficulty speaking and understanding others
- Numbness or paralysis of one side of the face, arm, or leg
- Blurred or doubled vision or temporary blindness
- A severe headache with dizziness or nausea
- Loss of balance and coordination
- Sudden loss of consciousness

Both the symptoms and the consequences of strokes are extremely frightening. About 1 in 3 strokes are fatal, 1 in 3 results in permanent, irreversible damage, and 1 in 3 have no lasting effects. Also, a mild stroke is a dangerous sign because it can lead to a series of future strokes.

A stroke is an emergency in which early action and immediate medical attention are crucial. Effective medical treatment can also prevent disability from stroke.

Type 2 diabetes: A disorder in which the pancreas stops producing insulin or does not use it properly. This leads to low absorption of glucose by the cells or by the liver that stores it. As a result, there is an increase in glucose levels in the blood and urine. People may be unaware of having this disorder because the symptoms develop slowly over the years. However, individuals who have type 2 diabetes usually overeat and are overweight.

Currently, about 1 in 3 adults have prediabetes. Early detection and proper treatment for this common ailment can decrease its severe complications, which include blindness, kidney failure, nerve damage, and heart disease, among others.

The symptoms of type 2 diabetes are:

- Frequent urge to urinate
- Being constantly thirsty
- Feeling hungry after eating
- Sudden weight loss
- Extreme fatigue and tiredness
- Slow healing of cuts and wounds
- Itching around the genitals
- Numbness, tingling, and pain in hands and feet
- Blurry vision

No matter where you are in diabetes 2 path, patients can achieve a total reversal with lifestyle changes. The recovery process starts with your learning to manage your disorder. You will also need to follow your doctor's advice, be tested, check your blood sugar regularly, lose weight, eat healthy foods, be active, and manage your stress.

Cancer: It is an uncontrolled growth and spread of abnormal cells. Cell division and growth are controlled by genes, which sometimes malfunction and cause damage to the body. Cell overgrowth can be benign, which is harmless, or malignant, which spreads to other tissues and organs. Malignant cells may be spread by the bloodstream or through the lymphatic system.

The invasion of healthy tissues by a malignant tumor is called metastasis. It takes about 10 years for a malignant tumor to develop and damage blood vessels, nerves, or organs. Once cancer has metastasized, it is usually incurable. However, adequate treatment can prolong and improve the life of a cancer patient. Treatment usually includes surgery, chemotherapy, radiotherapy, and palliative care.

These are the warning signs or symptoms of cancer:

- Extreme fatigue
- Significant unintended weight changes
- Eating problems such as lack of appetite, indigestion, discomfort, nausea, or vomiting
- A lump or swelling beneath the skin
- Skin changes such as sores, redness, darkening, growing moles, etc.
- Unusual bruising
- Blood in stools or urine
- Changes in bowel or bladder habits
- Vaginal bleeding
- Persistent coughing or trouble breathing
- Unexplained fever or night sweats
- Sudden vision or hearing problems
- Persistent muscle or joint pain
- Neurological problems, headaches, and seizures
- Major changes in the way your body works or feels

Cancer is the second cause of death worldwide, even though about 40% of cancers are preventable. Cancer is caused by gene mutations, viruses, and exposure to chemicals, tobacco, carcinogens, radiation, pollution, etc.

The best way to fight cancer is by preventing it or by detecting it before it fully develops or metastasizes. Some actions, such as keeping a healthy lifestyle or having regular checkups and screenings for early diagnosis, can decrease cancer risks significantly.

- It is always possible to adopt habits that reduce the devastating consequences of chronic diseases.

- A heart attack happens when the blood flowing to the heart is significantly reduced or blocked.

- Heart attacks and strokes are life-threatening emergencies that require immediate medical attention.

- Cancer is the second cause of death worldwide, even though many cancers are preventable.

Questions to reflect on:

1. Do you fear that any of your poor habits might lead to the development of a chronic disease? Explain

2. Are you aware of any genetic factors that can predispose you to develop a chronic disorder?

3. Based on the information in this chapter, are you at risk of developing Type 2 Diabetes?

4. Are you fully committed to the efforts required to improve your health?

Chapter 14:

Impact of the Environment on Our Health

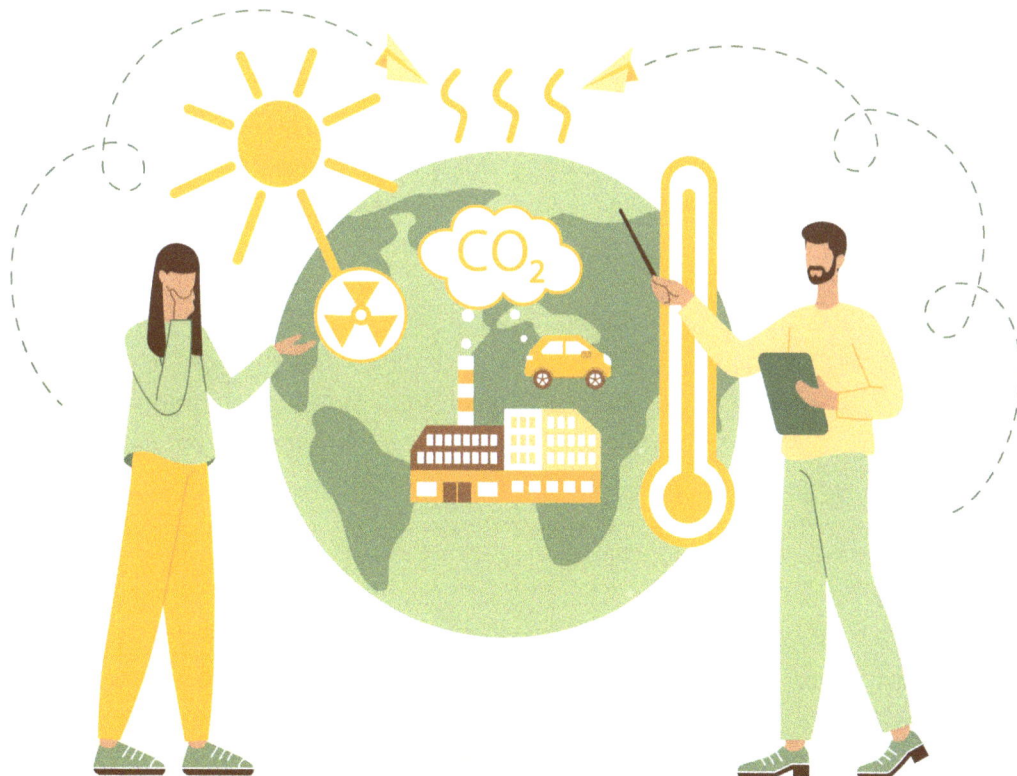

Responsible living to save our planet and ourselves

Our physical and mental health is directly related to the way we handle our individual space and our planet. The challenge of sharing the earth with 8 billion people forces each of us to reexamine the impact our actions and habits have on the environment.

We are being called to increase our environmental practices and acknowledge that our personal well-being and safety are tied to our common responsibilities to preserve our planet. Solving the global warming crisis demands individual and collective actions, lest we continue to experience significant human losses provoked by wildfires, hurricanes, floods, drought, rising seas, and other natural disasters, and an increase in infectious diseases.

Instead of falling into a state of environmental doom, feelings of despair, or climate anxiety, people might otherwise choose to take effective steps to engage in responsible stewardship of our planet. This is an urgent, doable endeavor that requires restorative solutions to prevent further ecological disasters. We have an obligation to preserve the extraordinary beauty of nature and the richness of resources.

In our large world, it is easy to assume that individual efforts to combat global warming have no major effects globally. However, we must not forget that the average person emits an average of 7 tons of CO_2 per year into the atmosphere. Thus, individual behaviors in relation to energy use, transportation, and consumption, contribute to carbon pollution.

People in developed countries have a larger carbon footprint than those in less developed nations, although the latter usually experience the most damaging consequences. Climate-related disasters increase poverty and human suffering when homes and critical infrastructure are destroyed, forcing large populations to migrate.

We all have the moral responsibility to prevent climate change by reducing our individual carbon footprint. We can no longer rely on governments to create policies that promote sustainable development and the use of resources to preserve our planet for future generations. Each of us should develop an awareness of how our own lifestyle can be modified to save our planet.

Given that each of us contributes to the problem of environmental pollution, we must also be part of the solution. To start, individual citizens can reduce their carbon footprint by committing to make smart choices in the use of energy, transportation, and food. They also need to modify their shopping habits.

The generation and consumption of energy have a direct impact on the environment, as it is in the case of fossil fuels. In contrast, electricity from renewable sources such as solar and wind do not cause greenhouse emissions or air pollution. Here are some recommendations for reducing energy use:

- Turning off lights and unplugging appliances when not in use
- Buying high-efficiency appliances and electronic products
- Using LED light bulbs
- Insulating homes to reduce energy for air conditioning and heating
- Adjusting thermostat settings to 78 degrees in the summer and 70 degrees in the winter
- Using cold water when doing laundry

Transportation is the leading cause of global warming worldwide. Cars, trucks, planes, ships, and trains release a significant number of pollutants into the atmosphere. Therefore, we must commit to taking steps to modify our transportation habits to reduce greenhouse gas emissions. To curb the damaging effects of transportation on climate, people can:

- Reduce the amount of time they spend driving and flying
- Take shorter trips and avoid layovers
- Use public transportation when possible
- Drive more fuel-efficient vehicles, keeping them in good condition
- Walk or bike if possible
- Carpool to work or use ride-sharing services
- Live closer to work or work from home if the job allows it

Along with energy reduction, water conservation is vital to environmental protection. Fresh, clean water is a limited resource and population growth puts extra pressure on its availability. Millions of people around the world do not have easy access to water; therefore, those who do must use it as efficiently as possible. Water-saving tips include:

- Being conscious of our individual water use and promoting water conservation
- Taking shorter showers
- Turning off the faucet when brushing our teeth or shaving
- Installing low-flow showerheads
- Checking and repairing water leaks
- Upgrading to Energy Star washing and dishwashing appliances
- Doing only full-load washes
- Using the dishwasher instead of washing dishes by hand
- Watering plants wisely

Our food choices and shopping habits also contribute greatly to air and water pollution. Therefore, adopting a more sustainable diet and responsible product consumption will help reduce our individual and collective carbon footprint.

From meat to vegetables, the growth, harvest, and distribution of food have adverse effects on the planet's ecosystems and biodiversity. It depletes natural resources and generates significant landfill waste. However, some foods cause more damage than others. For instance, livestock farming's greenhouse gas emissions are much higher than those related to the growth of fruits and vegetables. The following actions can help reduce our food carbon footprint:

- Buying less food
- Adopting zero-waste practices
- Controlling overeating
- Reducing meat consumption as much as possible
- Buying in-season fruits and vegetables
- Purchasing products with biodegradable packaging
- Avoiding items with individual-size packaging
- Storing food properly at home
- Donating excess food to food banks or other such organizations
- Always bringing reusable bags to the store when grocery shopping

While most people everywhere might be fond of shopping, few of us take time to consider the harmful implications of our buying habits. An increase in cheap products that are easily discarded further pollutes our environment. And obviously, the more goods we purchase, the larger the quantities that need to be manufactured.

In addition, the unprecedented growth of online shopping, or e-commerce, has started to have negative consequences on the environment. It is causing an even larger increase in greenhouse gas emissions than in-person shopping. When more parcels are packaged and shipped individually rather than in large-scale orders, they generate over-packaging waste and a staggering increase in transportation. Online purchasing has worsened shopping habits as large numbers of consumers request fast deliveries, which require even more energy use. Mindful, responsible, and ethical buying behaviors include:

- Being aware of our spending habits
- Becoming eco-conscious consumers
- Refusing plastic packaging, plastic bags, and plastic products
- Making purchases from environmentally friendly brands
- Changing the environmental practices of the industries we buy products from
- Buying from local resale businesses
- Reusing and recycling as often as possible
- Abstaining from impulse buying and purchasing only items that are needed
- Extending the lifespan of our possessions
- Repairing items that can be fixed instead of buying new ones
- Restraining from following fashion trends
- Home-cooking meals rather than ordering take out
- Avoiding any kind of waste and not choosing to shop as a form of recreation

Each of us is made accountable for fighting climate change. Our human response to the earth's well-being should be directly related to a curbing of our consumer obsession and an increase in environmental protection efforts. Reducing compulsive purchases is one of the best ways to improve our environmental habits because the less we buy, the kinder we are to our planet. Another is supporting entities and programs that promote sustainable lifestyles and build ecologically friendly societies.

Being mindful of the way our surroundings affect our well-being.

It is well-accepted that most people thrive in environments that are clean and well-organized because the organization and mental health go hand in hand. Overall, individuals who keep their homes and work areas tidy are more productive, happier, and healthier than those who do not. Dirty, cluttered spaces have a negative effect on our mental health; they usually affect our mood negatively, making us frustrated, anxious, and even depressed.

An orderly space makes us feel calm and balanced, increasing our sense of well-being. Simple actions like fixing our bed as soon as we get up every morning have the immediate effect of preparing us to tackle other daily responsibilities. As a child, I dreaded making my bed; I considered it a meaningless task until I came to realize that it was a very crucial habit to develop. In my experience, it has become the single most important factor that determines the quality of my day. This simple action gets me in a positive mood and strengthens my self-discipline at the same time.

The way we maintain our personal space can either promote healthy or unhealthy habits. Messy, dirty, and cluttered homes trigger negative behaviors. Thus, restructuring our environment while modifying behaviors is crucial to breaking bad habits and forming new ones. If you are on a path to healthier living, make sure that your new space favors achieving your objectives to improve your life and prevent repetitive actions that reinforce unhealthy behaviors.

An agreeable environment frees us to focus on what matters most. Living in a clean, well-scented home is liberating and makes it easier to be in control of our own actions. It contributes to reinforcing our motivation to undertake various challenges. In contrast, clutter and disorganization are stressors that generate mental chaos. It is virtually impossible to focus our attention on important tasks when we are surrounded by piles of clothes waiting to be put away or laundered and dirty dishes, among other things.

There is not a single approach to tidying up that suit everyone. Some people prefer to work on small areas little by little so that the task of organizing and cleaning does not become overwhelming. Other people choose to take a day or two and devote their energy to cleaning their homes and putting their personal items in order because that gives them a real sense of accomplishment.

Regardless of the strategy you choose, the following tips will help avoid the problem of environmental chaos:

Dispose of unnecessary items that take up space and make cleaning more difficult as you start decluttering.

Donate personal belongings that are usable but not essential to you. Having fewer possessions maximizes the living space in your home.

Develop a household organizational system that works well for your family, using as a guide "A place for everything and everything in its place."

Include cleaning routines in your weekly schedule and make them a priority.

Be consistent with your decluttering and cleaning. Don't allow things to get out of hand before choosing to get organized.

If you dislike cleaning or if it does not fit in with your regular routine, **hire someone** to perform that task for you.

Living in clean and tidy homes has great benefits for our health, such as:

- Improving sleep and rest
- Reducing stress, anxiety, and depression
- Improving interpersonal relationships
- Promoting the development of healthier habits
- Increasing positive attitudes and personal happiness

To keep in mind

- Individual behaviors in relation to energy use and transportation contribute greatly to carbon pollution.

- The unprecedented growth of online shopping has started to have negative consequences on the environment.

- Everyone is made accountable for fighting climate change.

- Most people thrive in environments that are clean and well-organized because organization and mental health go hand in hand.

- The way we maintain our personal space can either promote healthy or unhealthy habits.

Questions to reflect on:

1. Do you believe that individual efforts to prevent climate change can contribute to save our planet? Explain

2. What actions can you undertake to reduce your personal carbon footprint?

3. How does your personal space enhance or harm your physical or mental health?

4. What do you need to do to keep a tidier home?

www.ingramcontent.com/pod-product-compliance
Lightning Source LLC
Chambersburg PA
CBHW042346030426
42335CB00031B/3476

9 781959 670841